The Four Gifts
How One Priest Received a Second, Third, and Forth Chance at Life

By Father Joseph Bradley

Introduction by
Joseph F. Girzone

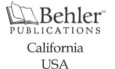

Behler™
PUBLICATIONS
California
USA

Behler Publications
California

The Four Gifts: How One Priest Received a Second, Third, and Fourth
Chance at Life
A Behler Publications Book

Copyright © 2013 by Joseph Bradley
Cover design by Yvonne Parks - www.pearcreative.ca.

Library of Congress Cataloging-in-Publication Data

Bradley, Joseph (Joseph P.)
  The four gifts : how one priest received a second, third, and forth [i.e. fourth] chance at life / by
Joseph Bradley.
     p. cm.
  ISBN 978-1-933016-75-7 (pbk.) -- ISBN 1-933016-75-2 (pbk.) 1. Bradley, Joseph (Joseph P.)--
Health. 2. Heart--Transplantation--Patients--California--Biography. 3. Priests--California--
Biography. I. Title.
  RD598.35.T7B73 2013
  617.9'54092--dc23
  [B]
                              2012030862

FIRST PRINTING

ISBN 13: 978-1-933016-75-7
e-book ISBN 978-1-933016-74-0

Published by Behler Publications, LLC
Lake Forest, California
www.behlerpublications.com

Manufactured in the United States of America

To my family,
for always believing

Table of Contents

Foreword

Fr. Joseph F. Girzone

Being a priest is a special calling. It is not something someone takes upon himself. The joys and honors are significant. The work is special in that it is totally focused on service, serving God and others, teaching, counseling, comforting, healing, being always there when needed, regardless of the time of day or night. There are no scheduled work hours. The task also entails listening endlessly to the pain in people's lives and offering hope in times of tragedy, and reconciling people to God when they come to him burdened with guilt. The most beautiful and humbling work of a priest is the honor bestowed on him by God; the power to gather his people together and present them to Jesus as He offers Him really and mystically to His Heavenly Father for the forgiveness of His people's sins, and the consecration of their lives. The work of a priest is closest to the life of Jesus, Himself, if the priest performs his ministry conscientiously.

When such a ministry is struck down early in life by a life-threatening illness, there is, obviously, a unique kind of heartbreak and tragedy. This book tells the story of a happy, conscientious, and dedicated young priest who loved his priesthood, loved the people he served, and the students he taught, and one day learned he did not have much time to live, and that his only hope was to have a heart transplant. The thought itself paralyzes one's ability to even think of such a future, much less a future in the stressful work of the priesthood.

This story tells in, a beautiful and inspiring way, how Father Joe Bradley faced this terrifying prospect and the drama of making a decision and living that decision with whatever time should remain in his life, and whether he would ever again be able to act out his sacred calling.

~ *Fr. Joseph F. Girzone*

Introduction

By all rights, knowledge, and plain old common sense, I should be dead. If past usage of beer, marijuana, and cocaine didn't do the trick, then certainly heart failure should have.

Instead, by the grace of God, I am alive, clean and sober, and a functioning Catholic priest. I'm not a survivor, I'm a miracle — the result of the remarkable power of prayer and faith in a mysterious, but loving and forgiving God, and a wonderfully supportive community. I needed both to survive addiction and the blessing of a heart transplant.

Gratitude inspired this book. I owe it to the people who helped rescue me from alcohol and drugs, and I owe it to my heart donor and family for giving me yet another chance at life. I owe it to my family for never giving up on me when they had every reason to do so. Lastly, I owe it to the doctors and staff at UCSF Medical Center for literally saving my life by performing a heart transplant when almost all hope was lost.

Yes, I owe a lot of people for the life I live today.

I wrote this book for those still out there whose lives have truly become unmanageable. I know what that's like, and I know how it feels. I also wrote for those languishing in bed in a hospital setting. I know that loneliness and frustration as well. I wrote this book for you…I wrote it for us.

Like you, I've had my share of challenges. My Dad died suddenly and unexpectedly when I was twenty years old. His loss devastated me. At the time, my response to emotional tension was to flee and seek refuge from the pain of reality. I found soothing, escapist bliss in a beer bottle and cocaine vial; they were my passion, and I pledged irrevocable devotion to both.

The slide into the abyss was ugly, and I only sought help when there was nowhere else to go. I had simply run out of options, and the game I played so well, and with such enthusiasm, was up.

Today my sobriety is pure grace. It humbled me and led me to want to serve others as a Catholic priest. But make no mistake about it, I don't see the world through the eyes of a clerical collar. Instead, I see it through the eyes of a former drunk and user. In fact, the day of my ordination as a priest, an old friend came to the Mass and announced for all to hear, "Well, now I can say I've seen a miracle."

I believe he was right.

For fifteen years, I functioned as a sober priest before my heart gave out from the same disease that killed my dad. Yet remarkably, another miracle came my way, and I was blessed to receive a new heart. During the most painful moment of their lives, an anonymous family gave permission to transplant the heart of their loved one into my body. I am profoundly grateful for the generosity from total strangers.

I count my blessings every day, every hour, every minute, every second. How many of us have received a second, third, and fourth chance at life? I have been granted the blessing of faith, sobriety, a new heart…a new life. I have been given much more than I deserve.

And so I offer this book as a testimony to what can happen when a confused and bitter young man opens his life and spirit and allows God and God's people to do for him what he simply could not do for himself.

~ *God Bless, Fr. Joe*

Prologue

August 5, 2005, 10:00A.M., Dr. Dana McGlothlin calmly walked into room 1024 in the Cardiac Unit of UCSF Medical Center, wearing a gentle smile, and looked me in the eye. She said the words I'd been waiting to hear for over a year: "We think we have a heart."

Her words didn't sink in right away. But on some level I must have understood because my heart went into overdrive. It started beeping like crazy, and we were quickly joined by a group of anxious nurses who'd been observing its output from the monitor at the main desk. Even Dr. McGlothlin looked concerned. "Joe, I need you to stay calm...try to relax."

Easier said than done.

After months of waiting and multiple surgeries on my deteriorating heart, I'd just been handed a miracle. A heart had been found that might actually be available for the transplant I needed to survive. I was alternately numb and ecstatic as I tried to take in the news. But calm? No way.

I did my best to fake it as Dr. McGlothlin assured me that the Medical Center's lead transplant surgeon was already consulting with doctors at another hospital to be sure this heart was a match for me. "We should know within the hour," she said, offering the same gentle smile, "but in the meantime, keep this to yourself because nothing is definite."

I confess that Dr. McGlothlin had barely made it into the hallway before I'd violated every one of her instructions. Grabbing the phone off the nightstand, I dialed my brother and sister, and then proceeded to call just about everyone I'd ever met in my life. "They might have a heart," I whispered again and again, to repeated shouts of joy.

Afterward, I settled back into the pillows on my hospital bed and tried to pray. By this point in my illness, I could no longer lie flat because the fluid buildup made it feel as if I were drowning. But that wasn't the only reason I struggled. Despite my renewed hope, I knew that in order for me to live, someone else had to die. Here I was, a forty-nine-year-old man with plenty of life behind me. What if my potential donor had children? What if he or she was a young person, someone whose life and dreams had just begun to unfold?

My frustration was compounded by the fact that I am a Roman Catholic priest. One might think that would have helped, but it only helped make me a lousy patient. Here I'd spent fifteen years sitting at bedsides just like mine, consoling the sick and the dying and yet, despite all the pat answers I'd doled out to others, I was unable to provide one for myself.

These feelings were interrupted a half hour later when Dr. McGlothlin returned. This time she was beaming from ear to ear. "It's perfect," she said. "It's a perfect match. The transplant team will be in to see you within the hour. You can call your family and friends with the good news."

I nodded sheepishly since the task had already been completed.

Sensing the calls had already been made, Dr. McGlothlin smiled and walked to the bed and hugged me, whispering, "Stay strong because we can do this."

I lost it.

Yep. Just cried a river as Dr. McGlothlin patted my shoulder and left the room.

Afterwards, I offered the first of many prayers for my donor. I thanked God for the remarkable chance to reclaim my life; actually to begin a new life with a new heart. I asked the Lord to bless the family of my donor as well…I couldn't imagine their courage and strength to offer someone else life during their darkest moment of grief.

And while I thanked God for the opportunity of new life, I also reflected on the life I had been given ….

Part 1
The First Gift: Reclaiming my Faith

1

Planting the Seeds

I'd always felt comfortable in church. It felt safe. I liked feeling the warmth of family and community gathered in prayer. The atmosphere was strong enough to conquer mind numbing homilies delivered by the vast majority of our parish priests. I looked forward to weekend Masses when young seminarians would visit the parish and break out their acoustic guitars and belt out some folk rock for the Communion meditation. I would reverently follow Mom and Dad to receive Holy Communion and walk back to my seat to the tune of Simon and Garfunkle's, "Homeward Bound." Dad would roll his eyes as the seminarian belted out verse after verse, while Mom would gently tug on his shoulder whispering something like, "Oh, John, relax, they mean well, and the kids like it."

Dad's roots were solidly grounded in the Latin Mass; he loved the majesty of the language and the formality of the liturgy. I think it's safe to say that guitars, holding hands while singing the Our Father, and top forty hits as recessional hymns were a tad bit challenging for him. But for me, it absolutely worked. It was soothing…even fun, and the seminarians seemed so real, like people we could actually talk to about the challenges of growing up in the mid-60s.

My Dad grew up with a completely different perspective of Church. He was raised in Kilsyth, a tough middle class town in Scotland, a hotbed of religious intolerance best defined by the never-ending battle between Catholics and Protestants. To this day, I remember Dad telling me that, as a child, he was taught (and resolutely believed) that Protestants were one step from hell from the moment of their conception. By direct contrast, Catholics held an uncommonly graced position in the Sacred Heart of Jesus. There was absolutely no room for middle ground. You were either in or out. Period. Amen. Alleluia.

I remember as a youngster asking how, simply walking the streets of Kilsyth, he could tell the difference between a Catholic and Protestant? "Simple," he replied, "It was all about the scarf you wore around your neck."

He was deadly serious.

It seems that scarf attire worn while attending a local soccer match was the visible mandate of all future destinies. A blue scarf depicted loyalty to the Protestant faith and fidelity to the local Ranger soccer team. By blessed contrast, a green scarf not only showed reverence to Holy Mother Church, but it also signified loyalty to God's privately owned soccer team:

Celtic United.

There it was: Good versus Evil.

Eternal life versus eternal damnation.

Nothing more and nothing less.

Dad would proudly tell me stories of roaming the streets of Kilsyth, "wearing the green" just daring the local Protestant "hoodlum" to look at him the wrong way. I sensed it was something of a rite of passage into Scottish manhood for many a young lad. The first time he defended the honor of his faith and battled with a Protestant was a mix of religious affiliation and/or un tempered zeal at a local soccer match.

Braveheart on the streets of Kilsyth.

Kick ass for Jesus.

To be honest, the image confused me because I couldn't figure how Jesus would somehow support an enthusiastic beat down in his name. Still, politics and global religious intolerance aside, I had great respect for Dad's commitment and devotion to his faith, and it was clearly the source of his strength. His faith was rigid and unyielding, but it defined his life and beliefs.

Dad wasn't one to shout his faith from the mountaintop, nor was he a man to offer an elegant reflection at a Sunday Mass or weekday church gathering. He lived his life simply, but with the highest of integrity. He walked the talk. He was generous to a fault and anyone down and out would find a sympathetic friend in Dad. When he offered himself in service, he did so without calling any unnecessary attention to himself. He saw Jesus as the living, breathing Source of his life. Dad's faith was devout and traditional, and he wouldn't have it any other way. I loved him for the man he was—honest, straightforward, and fearless.

But I do think we had different visions and interpretations of Jesus and his ministry. From my earliest days as a child, I saw Jesus as a wonderful, edgy radical with a passion to defend the outsider, the one who was lost. To me, he was the ultimate healer. He wasn't a Warrior God, he was a man of understanding and peace. I loved the complexity of His message and the fact that it was hard to grasp and even harder to live.

I admired the image of Jesus standing up to the authority figures of his day *demanding* that they care for the less fortunate. I loved that He was a troublemaker who had a soft heart for the lonely and those beaten down by life. I liked that He was fearless to challenge people to the demands of life in His kingdom. Even as a youngster, that was my attraction to Jesus. To me, He was the original countercultural rebel who stood defiantly against the social mores of His time. The love He preached was beyond radical. I mean it was flat out silly—"Love your enemies"—who lives like that? But that is what I genuinely respected about Him, and it was the image I brought with me to Catholic elementary and high school.

2
Catholic School

My initial image of Jesus as something of a long haired, wandering hippie, preaching selfless love to the tune of "Michael Row the Boat Ashore" was soon vanquished when I met the priests at St. Catherine's. They were a curious lot, to say the least.

Adorned daily in formal clerical collar and black suit, they were men of mystery. As youngsters in grammar school, we didn't know a thing about them. Other than a quick wave of the hand (while not breaking stride), they rarely interacted with us. We saw them at Mass and behind a screen in the Confessional, but that was about it. They were a total mystery to much of the school community.

However, each semester, Father would dramatically enter our classroom on Report Card Day. It was a monumental event. We would immediately rise to our feet when he entered the room and Sister, the person who actually taught the class, introduced him with equal reverence. Father would glance at each card and offer a brief social and theological commentary before calling each boy or girl to the front of the class to receive his or her grades. If the student received a low grade in conduct, they were met with a dramatic stare down, much like two boxers receiving instructions from the referee while staring at each other before the first bell. Intimidation was the order of the day, and Father always won. Who could compete with an adult male dressed in black who offered a commentary that included insights shared in Latin?

We were taught that Father took the place of Jesus at our liturgies. If that was the case, well, Jesus was quite a bit more authoritative than I'd initially imagined. We were flat out afraid to breathe at Mass, except to answer the prayers in a timely manner. I never really gave priesthood much of a thought during my elementary years of Catholic education. I sensed that the priests in black suits were somewhat removed from the altruistic and charismatic Jesus, who captured my imagination as a youngster.

All that changed when I entered Serra High School and sat in the classroom of Fr. John Kelly. He was a genuine maverick and years ahead of his time. He brought the Jesus I loved home to all of his students. The radical Jesus in jeans and T-shirt suddenly reappeared with passion and a thirst for social justice and peace.

Our theology class wasn't lecture, it was discussion. Fr. Kelly would weave stories of Vietnam, Kent State, and Watergate into our consciousness, then he'd lower his glasses to peer out and ask, "Just what do you think this crazy Jewish carpenter is thinking about all this?"

All of a sudden my original image and attraction to Jesus was resurrected before me. Fr. Kelly offered a portrait of Jesus that was dramatic and inspiring. I was taken in by his presentations. Jesus' vision of faith was grounded in action—Praxis—as opposed to short-term memorization of prayers.

In Fr. Kelly's vision, Jesus was more interested in the work of peace and justice than he was in well coordinated liturgical services. That was news to many of us.

I was never comfortable or impressed with those who dressed in the finest of priest vestments for Mass, then put me to sleep in their homilies. But I was totally moved by those involved in the community. From as far back as I can remember, I admired the priests who stood up for the poor and walked in marches for peace.

In fact, I was so moved by the vision of priesthood that Fr. Kelly offered during my senior year, I seriously considered applying to the seminary. I wanted to be like the brave priests Fr. Kelly described—the ones who stood up to racism and sexism, and worked for full scale integration throughout our land—priests like Jesus, who were fearless to rock the boat in pursuit of justice.

I felt being a priest would give real meaning and purpose to my life. As an introvert and a quiet, shy kid, I basically hid in the shadows throughout high school. I probably uttered less than a hundred words in class the entire four years. I had lots of friends and was respected and liked by my classmates, but I was definitely one of those kids on the outer edge of the social hierarchal structure. At home, I realized that I wasn't the athlete my brother was, or the natural leader my sister was; I was simply your basic "Joe," a decent young man with good grades, who was just beginning the search for meaning in my young life.

Church was the place I always felt most safe and confident. It was the one place I was completely at ease with myself. I know this may sound terribly naïve, and even theologically inaccurate, but I think I saw priesthood as a safe, protective womb from the challenges and struggles of life. I'd be so busy doing good things for people that I'd miss the messiness of life, even the pain of life. I think there was a not-so-subtle sense of escapism mixed with a rather romantic feeling that it was entirely honorable to leave the world in pursuit of a higher calling.

Like most teenagers, I think I had this deep pathological need to feel safe and protected, and service in the Church community seemed to provide both.

It felt like entering a sanctuary where people shared a commonality of spiritual growth and service. Participating in liturgies and helping on youth retreats felt "home" to me, and it was where I thrived and felt fulfilled. It was where I was truly comfortable and happy. I wanted to make it my life's work.

That deep-seated feeling of needing safety even applied to relationships with girls in the neighborhood. Like all teenagers, I had felt rejection from more than one girl, but rather than stick to it and try again, I thought it made more sense to simply head off in a totally different direction. I would succeed in offering good service to people while, at the same time, avoiding emotional pain from future personal relationships. In effect, I was taking myself out of the game, but for a most worthy cause. At least that's how I justified it at the time.

I saw myself participating in a vibrant and caring ministry, while living in a protective shell far removed from the pressures and wounds of daily life. Bottom line: Priesthood was an honorable path, and one that offered a seal of protection from personal hurts and disappointments, and perceived or imagined failures. In addition, it was clear to me that people loved their priests. They spoke of them in glowing terms and honored their commitment to God. Deep down, I found that equally attractive.

Thus, for me, it was the perfect setup. I could devote myself to good works, miss out on the grittiness of life, and have people believe I was special for doing the work of God.

It wasn't until years later, on the verge of graduating from seminary, that I realized such a perspective was actually a cowardly choice. It was selfish and rooted more in self-preservation than actual service to the larger community. Today, I find it thoroughly embarrassing, but I can rationalize my emotions by admitting they were the thoughts and feelings of a seventeen year old.

But at the time, it made impeccable sense, so, I made up my mind to talk to Mom and Dad about applying to the college seminary.

I was surprised at their response. They both felt it was important to "live a little" before beginning the process. They encouraged me to attend a secular college, buy a car, and date more girls. Then, if I still wanted to apply, I could with their complete support. It was the kind of level, steadfast response so typical of my folks.

With some reluctance, I accepted their wisdom. (Today, over thirty years later, most major seminaries will offer the same advice to aspiring seminarians—experience life with all its joys and pitfalls, then if you still feel the call, you may apply.)

While attending a local junior college and working part-time loading bags and cleaning planes at a major airline at the San Francisco Airport, I made visits to church several times a week. I would snuggle into a pew somewhere in the middle of the church and lose myself in prayer.

I had absolutely no desire to join the work crew for a few beers after work, nor did I have any desire to attend their parties. I was friendly with all of them and genuinely liked working with them, but my heart and sights were set in a very different direction.

What was prayer at that time? I think it was a conversation where I did most of the talking. It was like having a diary of thoughts without writing anything down. It was free-fall, helter-skelter of whatever thought or emotion entered my mind. Sadly, there was almost no room for listening—at least on my part. I would pour my heart out to my "Counterculture Peacenik Jesus" who knew my joys and sorrows and was ready to open the door to his seminary, so I could keep his message of peace and justice alive.

I never slowed down or paused to sit quietly and allow my thoughts to breathe in union with the Lord's spirit. No, this was more like bringing a specific agenda of where I wanted to go and hoping the good Lord would grant my wish. Looking back, I can see that while well intentioned, it was a remarkably immature form of prayer. It lacked humility. It lacked the awareness and discipline to quietly consider exactly what the Lord wanted for me because I was too busy asking Him to grant my wish, on my terms, in a timely manner. I thought I had my future all mapped out and ready to go.

3

The Shock of Sudden Death

I think it was John Lennon who once sang, "Life is what happens while you're busy making other plans." My favorite Beatle had it right.

While I was busy making other plans to enter the seminary and become a priest, the damndest, most unexpected thing happened: Dad died.

The Rock. The solid backbone of our family and for many in the local community was gone at the ridiculous age of fifty-one.

Unbeknownst to anyone, including himself, Dad's heart had been in failure for a long time. He was a lifelong smoker and we had noticed his recent lack of stamina and the ferocious morning cough for several months. His doctor was concerned but never actually sat down and explained the seriousness of the diagnosis: dilated cardiomyopathy—a disease that destroys the heart muscle, causing it to swell as it ceases to pump oxygen throughout the cardiovascular system. There is no cure. In fact, the only way to survive is to receive a heart transplant.

Dad was on a business trip to Greenville, Pennsylvania, when he developed another cold that quickly settled into pneumonia. With his heart significantly weakened, he simply could not fight off the infection, and he died, March 2, 1978.

The shock was immeasurable for all of us. Mom literally guided my sister, Maureen, brother, Johnny, and I through Dad's funeral. For me, it was a major turning point in my spiritual journey because the spiritual journey ended the moment Dad died. It was the start of a downfall that lasted several years and hurt a lot of people, including myself.

I felt betrayed when Dad died, and I was more than a little angry with God.

My kindhearted, gentle, Jesus had let me down. I remember walking down a long hallway in the last hours of Dad's life and slipping into a tiny room marked with a sign that said, "Quiet."

Hoping for a few quiet moments of prayer, I distinctly remember thinking that one of the most attractive things about Jesus' life was His unique ability to heal and reconcile. My faith taught me that He was capable of restoring life to those who called on Him with a sincere heart.

I also remember being taught in elementary school by the Sisters of Mercy that whatever we asked of God — *if* we asked with a pure heart, it would be granted. The wonderful and dedicated sisters assured us that God would always help us, and went to great lengths to promise that God loved us so dearly that we could always count on Him.

Well, here I was asking for God's help, and I was counting on Him to respond. I remember kneeling on the hard marble floor of the chapel and saying, "Heal this good and holy man, Lord, and I will be your priest forever."

At that moment, there was nothing altruistic or spiritual about my promise to be a priest; it was a flat out bargain. It was a deal between a desperate young man and the Almighty. Heal Dad and I'll enter the seminary in short order. I looked at my offer as something of a payback for a deed well done. It was a win-win situation: Dad gets restored to health, and God gets a priest. It was meant as a simple and direct bargain where everyone gets what they want. I thought it was perfect.

I left the meditation room with no doubt that Dad would be healed momentarily. I half expected to see him sitting up in a chair asking Mom what she was so worried about. But when I entered his room, it was Mom sitting in the chair practically convulsing with tears that told me he was gone. Without anyone saying a word, I knew this was a catastrophe. The doctor came over and put his arm around my twenty-one-year-old shoulder and said as much. "Joe, I am so sorry, but your father is gone."

I must have looked at him with a blank stare, because he repeated it, "I am sorry, Joe, but your dad has died."

I still could not comprehend what he was saying, but Mom's sobbing cleared any doubt. My legs gave way and, without realizing it, I fell to the floor. I sat on the floor next to the bed and stared at nothing and no one. The doctor and nurse helped me to my feet and for the first time I made eye contact with Dad's lifeless body. I saw suffering in his face. It all seemed so brutal.

I remember excusing myself and walking back to the meditation room I had just left moments ago. I looked down at the rosary beads I carried with me to the hospital and a St. Jude prayer card someone must have given to me before we left California.

Entering the chapel, I said, "Jesus, you let me down—how could you do this? In our darkest moment of need, I believe you walked away from us, and I don't think I can ever trust you again. You could have helped and chose not to—which is bad—or you *couldn't* help—which is worse. Either way, you disappeared, and I am way beyond disappointed. I will never forget this day or moment of your betrayal."

For me, it was a clear violation of everything I had been taught as a child and young man. Until that moment, I believed God would make all things right if we just asked with a pure, humble heart.

Bullshit.

That's not what happened.

My words and emotions were all about hurt and betrayal. Lost in the anger and outrage were the twelve years of planting the seeds of faith evaporating within seconds of the first test. It is sad to admit, but when Dad died that cold March afternoon, my faith died with him. The seeds of faith were uprooted through the sorrow of loss. It took all of a minute to turn my back on everything I was taught to believe.

On the way out of the hospital, Mom lost her footing and slipped on the cold cement. I picked her up with one arm and supported her with the other. As we walked to the car, I noticed a trash can and casually flipped my rosary beads and St. Jude card into it, where they found a home with all the other trash. At the time, I thought it was an entirely appropriate action.

4

Rebellion

The irony never occurred to me that in less than three months before Dad's death, I was all set to apply to seminary to become a Catholic priest. But my first taste of sorrow and loss destroyed any thought of applying. The "safety and protection" I saw in religious community was shattered and with it my hopes of becoming an ordained minister. It was an important lesson to realize that nothing in life is perpetually safe and protected. Just because one wears a religious habit does not make the person immune to the sorrows of life.

Still, even I was surprised at how quickly my faith disintegrated. Within moments after the doctor declared the official time of Dad's death, I no longer considered myself Catholic...or anything else for that matter. Obviously, the seeds of my faith were not planted on solid ground. Jesus may have encouraged his disciples to build their faith on sturdy rock, but mine was clearly built on mushy sand. It didn't survive the test, and it opened the door to some seriously self-destructive behavior.

Dad's funeral Mass was a major community event. The church was packed and several priests manned the altar, while I sat in the front row sharing small talk with my younger brother. The only reason I went to communion was to not hurt Mom or insult our extended family, many of whom traveled a long way to be part of the Mass.

I went back to work the next day. Gone were the days of stopping off at church on the way home for a few moments of prayer. I put college on hold and consciously decided to embrace life at the airlines where free flight passes awaited with promises of good times.

Mom was only forty-eight at the time of Dad's death, and her faith astounded me. To the core of her being, she believed Dad was with her in a new spiritual way each and every day of her life. Mom would frequently visit church and light candles to his memory and arrange Mass intentions in his name.

Her oldest son was determined to follow a very different path.

I turned my back on everything I'd been taught to believe in as a child. Looking back, I thing that, deep down, I wanted to hurt God, and His Son, and His Spirit. I wanted to disappoint him. I wanted to change the direction of my life.

I wanted to hurt God by violating every sacred tenet I had been taught. Now, the fact that such behavior would only lead to hurting me simply went unnoticed because I was too deep in grief and rage to see the larger picture.

I never drank much alcohol in high school. Simply put, I didn't like it, and I didn't like what it did to people. I preferred an occasional taste of marijuana and was way more comfortable with its calming sensation than the uninhibited chaos of alcohol. Under the influence of alcohol, my high school pals changed and became highly aggressive, and I wasn't comfortable watching the evolution. But marijuana was different; after a few tokes from a bong, the only thing we fought about was who would get the first Twinkie or cupcake.

But in the months following Dad's death, I began to snuggle up to a cold beer to take the edge off everything related to grief. It wasn't long before a pattern began to emerge: a few beers in a quiet setting soon became several, which soon became a lot, which all led to a sense of liberation from the emotional pain. I wasn't a big party drinker; I was much more a solitary drinker—to quote the great rocker George Thorogood, "I Drank Alone."

My instinct for dealing with emotional stress has always been to flee. I think there is a part of me that *wants* to confront the pain, but there's a much larger part that simply wants to run away and pretend it's not there. Beer and the occasional shot of Mr. Daniels became a soothing balm for escape. Almost without realizing it, using alcohol began to take on a life of its own, one that would progress from enjoyment, to passion, to obsession. I liked the quick, soothing sensation I received from a beer or shot of whiskey. It served to temporarily absorb some of my stress and depression over losing Dad.

As for God and faith, my relationship with the Lord had gone way past hurt and disappointment, and had settled in the sanctuary of perpetual bitterness and cynicism.

The sad part is I actually began to *like* how it felt. I actually liked feeling angry and bitter. It became something of a vicious loop; the more I drank, the more bitter I became, and the more bitter I became, the more I drank. It was a crazy cycle, but not crazy enough to make me want to jump off.

Why did my faith fall apart so quickly? I think part of the problem was that I brought a huge sense of entitlement to all matters of God, faith, and Church. Somewhere beneath the altruistic call to serve was an inherent need to experience the payoff. And for me, the payoff was a smooth-sailing, hassle-free life, and the respect of the larger community. I'd believed that devoting my life to Church and Faith meant having a life without conflict. It simply never occurred to me that *real faith* meant having a sense of internal peace *within* the conflict.

I think I had this impression that working for the Lord somehow entitled me to freedom from the normal pains of life. So when tragedy and sorrow raised its ugly head, I was completely unprepared to handle it. Alcohol was the nearest and quickest means to subjugate the pain, so I dove in, even though I knew it was, at best, a temporary solution.

5

High Times at the San Francisco Airport

In the late '70s and early '80s, many airlines began hiring young employees as the San Francisco Airport expanded its service. It was an exciting time to be in the airline industry. Given the times, it's fair to acknowledge that drug and alcohol use was quite prevalent throughout the industry. It was such a different culture from present-day life at the airport. Like me, my airline pals were all in their early twenties with their entire lives just beginning to unfold, and we took our travel and partying very seriously.

Between denying God, my father's death, and my daily life with alcohol, I brought a major chip on my shoulder to work each day. I didn't even care that I was hurting myself. I developed an angry 24/7 persona that would not yield an inch.

God was for weaklings, and His church was for the weakest of the weak. I mocked it. I taunted it in my mind while gleefully breaking every commandment I could think of, going so far as actually go out of my way to do things that violated every law I'd been taught to obey.

Ironically, in the wild days of the late '70s, such recklessness actually inspired new friendships among the work crew. We were young and strong and (seemingly) free to push our lives to the limit, and I threw myself into the process with focused devotion and zealous enthusiasm.

Most of the new employees were my age, and several of us knew each other from high school. Going to work was like going to a party—full of laughter and good times. Alcohol and marijuana were liberally shared, as was the custom of the time, and our entire culture revolved around our use of drugs.

Each month, we would dutifully board a plane in the morning for a scheduled "road trip." At the airline's expense, we would fly off to Atlanta or Jacksonville and take in a rock concert with the likes of Aerosmith or Lynyrd Skynryd topping the bill. After an evening of alcohol-fueled fun, we would grab a few hours of sleep on the flight home and return to work the following day. I had an absolute blast constantly trying to outdo the hijinks of the previous trip.

Beer and marijuana were the staples of each trip. Of course, in those days, you could simply walk to the boarding area with baggage in hand, so as airline employees, our bags were never even checked. Thus, I would stroll onto the plane with hefty amounts of marijuana safely tucked into my overnight bag, and no one knew or suspected a thing. We were all amazed at our good fortune.

I was delighted to find an excellent source for high grade marijuana at the airport through a nice guy who worked on the grounds. He'd arrive at work each day with nickel and dime bags tucked inside his gym bag, so we welcomed him as an extended member of our work crew, and would rotate purchasing a few of the bags every night. Less than an hour after arriving at work at least half the crew was high. Even though I was having a ball, I sensed that alcohol and marijuana were slowly taking over all phases of my life. While I was never out of control high or drunk, I was never actually sober, either. I would nurture a nice, lazy high all day and float from one adventure to another.

One day while working at the airport cleaning and loading planes, a friend came over during a break, and said, "Joe, are you OK? You look really tired."

"Yeah, I'm fine, just relaxing before the next flight arrives," was my less than enthusiastic response.

"Come with me, I've got something that will sharpen you up in no time at all."

Together we strolled into an empty room near the main office where the pilots and flight attendants gathered to receive flight plans before boarding the plane. Since the room was empty, we locked the door and settled at an empty table where my co-worker reached into her pocket and pulled out a tiny vial filled with white powder.

"What is it?" I woke up to ask.

"It's cocaine—you will *love it*—heck, you'll be wide awake and rolling in a minute."

"Let's do it," I said, leaping at the new opportunity.

The vial had a tiny, elegant spoon attached, and she dug out a healthy amount and suggested I snort it. I thought the whole scene was rather seductive, enchanting—there was an element of danger to it that I found irresistible. Where marijuana seemed giddy and harmless, cocaine had a dark quality to it.

I absolutely loved it. It was to become my new life partner.

From the first moment it slid down my nasal cavity I knew I was in for the long haul. I wanted more before finishing the first spoonful. Soon, there was no getting enough, and it didn't take long to develop an obsession with the drug.

I loved the physical rush of adrenaline and the sense of emotional euphoria. All of a sudden, I could talk to beautiful women without avoiding direct eye contact. Hell, I felt damn near omnipotent and fearless. The shift wasn't half over when I was asking where I could purchase some more. To my surprise, I learned that for a mere $25.00 I could buy a quarter gram from the same man who was selling us marijuana at work.

It was beautiful.

I would usually start each shift with a toke of marijuana in my car, then once I arrived at work, I would wash it down with a cold one. As the shift moved along and things began to get a little sloppy, I would switch over to cocaine to sharpen up so I could go out and enjoy a few beers at the end of the day.

And that was a typical workday. Days off were simply a blur.

Thirty years later, it sounds ludicrous to admit how cocaine seemed to fill that old emotional need to feel safe. And I did, indeed, feel safe under its influence. I had that same feeling of acceptance and joy I had as a youngster at church—that's how deep it went. Because drug use was so much part of the culture in the late '70s and early '80s, I never gave a thought to consequences.

The work crew became like a big extended family, and we attended each other's family evens, and reached out to each other in times of trouble or crisis. We were never without marijuana or coke. I even shared it with one of my bosses. He was a good hard-working guy, and I was happy to share. Besides, I thought it might be good for my own security. Nothing like dealing and sharing coke with one of the people responsible for my evaluation.

But under the almost daily influence of cocaine, alcohol, and marijuana, my pals and I soon slipped into new and deeper manners of recklessness at work. I began stealing liquor off arriving flights. As luck would have it, one of my assigned tasks was to count and record the number of used liquor bottles stored in the lower compartments of the airplane after it landed.

Hard to believe, right? The powers that be actually assigned that responsibility to *me*. Of course, I graciously accepted it with eyes aglow at future possibilities.

As soon as the plane landed and the passengers departed, I would board and quickly make a beeline to the belly of the plane where the liquor cabinets were stored.

Arriving at the galley, I would munch on a stale sandwich and wash it down with a semi-cold beer. I would load the liquor cases onto a truck and drive over to the liquor room, ironically located next to the personnel office.

Once inside the liquor room, I would open the containers with a key and search for the recording log, which gave an account of the bottles used during the flight. I would then make several "adjustments" to the original count. So if six bottles of Jack Daniels were used, it quickly became nine. After an hour or so, I'd assembled a lovely mix of drinks, which I graciously shared with the crew during our break.

I even had a lookout watching the liquor room door to alert me if one of the lead agents was in the vicinity. Tony Soprano would have blushed at my brazen willingness to lift everything in sight. I even stole extra beer and wine from the First Class section; I would hide the bottle in a large shopping bag and drive out to the parking lot to store them in my trunk to enjoy with the crew after work.

Looking back, I realize how completely rudderless I was. Without a sense of faith in my life, there was no core, no center. Life was all about the rush, and I flew from one thing to another without thought, reflection, or care. I didn't want to slow down because it might mean confronting how I was living. I preferred full throttle with no sense or desire to look back.

But despite the multiplicity of drugs slithering through my system on a 24/7 basis, I still wasn't happy, and I still wasn't at peace. In fact, it was getting worse. I was losing control. I started acting more reckless at home and at work. And still, despite what was becoming a clear, unquestionable fact that I had a real issue with drugs and alcohol, and my life was spinning out of control, I refused to give in. I was locked in a battle with the Lord as to who could hurt whom. I was determined to have careless fun, and damn the consequences.

Not that people didn't try and convince me to change my ways. Mom spoke with me every chance she could, and my sister took me out to lunch and dinner many times to offer her concerns. Even my brother, nine years younger than I, spoke from his heart, and nothing got through. I believed I was having fun. Though I knew I was playing with fire and heading full-tilt toward disaster, I still thought I could control my drinking and using, and even make it work.

Perhaps, the most infamous—and reckless—story of life at the airline was the night one of the employees actually came to work bearing homemade brownies to celebrate my upcoming birthday. They were lovingly sprinkled with marijuana and were liberally shared with most of the crew during our break. They were just lovely with a hot cup of coffee (touched up with a little Jack Daniels); soothingly satisfying the palate and calming the mind in such a manner that several employees (including me) sampled more than one of the delicacies. Little did we know or care that marijuana, ingested in such a manner, goes directly into the bloodstream and has a rather instant and dramatic effect on one's central nervous system. When our break was over, the crew stumbled through a rousing rendition of Happy Birthday...and immediately faded into oblivion.

I was frozen in time and space.

I could neither move nor speak.

In fact, the only physical gesture I could make was to fall over laughing at absolutely nothing.

However, moments later, I recovered enough to hop into a truck and navigate it towards *a multibillion dollar aircraft* that had just landed. Although I was driving no more than ten miles-per-hour, it felt like being on the front seat of a ride at Great America.

Deep down, we all knew this couldn't last forever; it just simply couldn't go on without a price to pay.

The downfall began when a lead agent asked to speak with me privately, away from the crew. He was a caring man who was genuinely concerned about my behavior and simply wanted to talk about what he suspected was going on with the crew. I would have none of it and was uncooperative. Sensing my unwillingness to give an inch, he became frustrated and stated that the previous month's liquor inventory showed a *remarkable* upswing of alcohol use on several arriving flights. In fact, it was so remarkable that he was beginning to wonder if we might be dealing with employee theft. He sternly advised that I should keep a close eye out to ensure that no one went near the liquor cabinets without express permission from one of the lead agents. I looked him in the eye with the devotional spirit of an altar boy and assured him that is exactly what I planned to do, adding for dramatic, albeit mocking emphasis, "Gee, this is terrible, I mean theft is a sin."

I never blinked and said it with a straight face.

6

Investigation: Corporate Security

As the late George Harrison once wrote, "All Things Must Pass," and although I didn't realize it, that meeting with the lead agent spelled the beginning of the end. It also instigated a monumental spiritual showdown between the good Lord and His wayward son. If I had doubted Jesus' healing presence, I would soon beg Him to reveal Himself. My "bottom" was fast approaching, and it would prove to be an ugly, costly fall from what remained of my integrity and grace. I was about to hit my knees.

Much to my surprise, not everyone was enamored with the youthful indiscretions of the evening work crew. A veteran employee had simply had enough. He was appalled that a bunch of twenty-something kids were stealing liquor, smoking dope, and snorting cocaine while on duty. He also found it highly offensive that we were putting ourselves and others in danger driving around the concourse, wreaking havoc with enough chemicals on board to feed a small army. My thoughts at the time? The poor old guy needed to get more fun out of life. He was taking the whole thing much too seriously.

But if I was determined to raise hell with complete disregard to basic rules of respect, he was equally determined to bring things to a thundering halt. Ultimately, his response to our (my) behavior was to write a long and remarkably detailed letter to the corporate security office. It spoke of rampant theft, alcohol and drug use, and general disregard for all issues of safety. He also suggested that the leading culprit was yours truly.

Within days, I learned that the airline was sending a corporate security officer to investigate the situation in San Francisco, and the person they most wished to speak with was me. A close friend called and said, "Off the record, Joe, they know everything, and they want your head on a platter."

So what was my first response? What did I do knowing full well that my job was in jeopardy? Yep, I stayed true to form and looked for a place to hide within myself by firing up a bong, drinking a cold beer, and slipping blissfully off to sleep.

I would literally go to any length to avoid facing reality, preferring to burrow into my own darkness, which I somehow found tranquil. The darker and more sullen things appeared to be, the more I relaxed and retreated within myself. It's easy to see now that my behavior was just the saddest kind of loneliness, and that I was walking a path that led to a dead end.

The following morning, I parked in the employee parking lot to catch the bus to the ramp area. Just before getting on, I pulled a small vial from my pocket and snorted a spoonful of cocaine to insure a pleasant, confident manner during my little chat with the security agent. At this point, I was totally dependent on chemicals to lift my mood and temperament. Since I no longer prayed or did much inner reflection, I counted on a mix of chemicals to carry the moment. It never occurred to me that, under the circumstances, the agent might ask for an *immediate* blood test.

When I arrived at the employee break room, the department manager pulled me aside and gently said, "Joe, there is a guy here from corporate security who has traveled a long way to speak with you."

Still buzzing euphorically, I smiled and nodded, "Let's go see The Man."

Thirty years later, I still remember his name was Dave. I was escorted into a room where the windows had been taped over with white paper to meet the rather imposing figure of Agent Dave. Ironically, it was the same room where I first tried cocaine.

There was a complete absence of small talk as Agent Dave immediately stated his purpose for flying out to San Francisco. He reminded me of Sgt. Joe "Just the Facts" Friday, from the old TV show *Dragnet*. While his head moved back and forth, his shoulders remained square and tight as he bluntly asked about drinking and drug use during work hours.

I offered my best, "Let's be pals" smile and denied everything. Then, as the cocaine rattled through my system, I offered, "Gee, Dave, I'm really hurt by this, I mean, your question almost seems like an accusation."

He asked if I was aware of anyone in the department using or dealing drugs during work hours. Of course, I looked at him blankly and shook my head. "No."

My entire demeanor was one of disrespect. I walked in with coke buzzing through my brain and acted like a bitter, angry kid who would not be intimidated. I was melting away from the young man I used to be, and had become quite successful in rejecting everything I was taught to believe.

I think Agent Dave sensed that the twenty-something kid sitting defiantly in front of him was fighting a war on many fronts, and he wasn't as tough as he made out to be. Near the end of the meeting, he pushed his paperwork aside, leaned back in his chair, and looked me in the eye. "Look, Joe, I have talked with your bosses and they've told me you're a hard working young man who has gone through a tough time, and they want to help you...so I want you to tell me the truth about what is going on, and I'll help. But once you leave this office, I will begin a thorough investigation, and I'll find out, and then I will come after you. This is your one and only chance to come clean with me."

I remember thanking him, and mumbling something about "everything was fine."

Oh hell yeah, everything was just fine and dandy.

I was up to my eyeballs in beer, marijuana, and cocaine, and my employer was on the hunt to have me fired...but yeah, everything was fine. No sense looking at reality.

The sad truth is that the only thing the investigation did was move everything underground; that is, my core group of friends and I became much more careful about our activities at work. I continued to steal liquor from arriving flights, but we were much more careful and less brazen in our activities.

There was one thing Agent Dave did leave me with; a subtle but very real sense of impending doom. I couldn't explain it, but I couldn't deny it either. There was a tangible sense that disaster was in the air. It was stronger than a premonition, and I was certain something terrible was going to happen...and happen soon. I just knew we would all pay a severe price for our collective behavior.

7

Steve Olsen

My friendship with Steve Olsen changed the course of my life.
Not even a corporate investigation could accomplish what Steve
did.

Steve joined the airline during a lull after the investigation. A
recent transfer from Boston, Steve was more than six feet tall, with
long brown hair. He was a former high school star quarterback with
a refreshingly uninhibited sense of humor. He was an instant hit
with everyone, especially the ladies. Many of the guys, including
me, would attach ourselves to Steve at various airline events—not
because he asked or invited us—we were just hoping to tag along in
the hope of meeting one of the girls he discarded, or simply left
behind.

Steve fit in with our little motley night work crew. One night
during a break, we agreed to meet the following morning for some
basketball—it was a week before Good Friday. The fact that it was
Lent, on the verge of Holy Week, meant absolutely nothing to me. It
was just a chance to play some ball before coming into work.

The following morning, Steve, a close pal, Kenny Romes, and I
gathered on a gorgeous spring morning in Menlo Park to play a few
hours of some serious hoops. Steve brought an old buddy from
Boston, and it was their plan to "school" the West Coast lads on the
finer points of basketball. Steve was a serious and successful athlete,
and we had no hope of stopping him...a fact he reminded us
throughout the game.

I remember talking briefly about the investigation before
dropping it all together. I brought the conversation to a close by
saying, "Look, fellas, this will pass. We need to just shut the hell up

and stonewall their questions. Speaking of which, I took the liberty to load a pipe for our post game celebration."

Everyone laughed, and we blocked everything else out and set out to enjoy some basketball on a gorgeous spring morning. After a few hours, we stopped for lunch at one of the local pubs in Palo Alto and shared some laughs over several beers. A short time later, we left in search of a sports bar to catch some more basketball, as well as the beginning of Spring training baseball games. I remember Kenny and I engaging Steve in a spirited dialogue on the natural superiority of West Coast athletics. Steve would have none of it, passionately remaining true to his love for the Celtics, Patriots, and Red Sox.

It was pure innocence. We were just four young guys shooting the bull about sports over some beers after a few hours of basketball. Eventually, we made our way to a park and took in the sun while making plans to visit Boston and catch a Red Sox game. Of course, we picked up an additional six pack and shared beers as the morning slowly evolved into late-afternoon.

I remember reaching into my gym bag and pulling out the pipe, which we shared as the laughs and jokes kept coming. At a certain point, I began to feel tired and sloppy and, realizing it was time to get ready for the ride home, I pulled a small vial of coke out of the same bag and passed it around to anyone willing to partake of its blessings. Cocaine had long been my remedy to emerge from a highly advanced marijuana stupor.

Moments later it was time to say our goodbyes and head home for some sleep before coming into work for the night shift. I remember looking at Steve and whispering, "Let's all drive carefully, and I'll see you guys tonight, so we can plan the trip to Boston." Steve smiled as he climbed into the passenger seat...and, in an instant, was gone.

When I arrived at work that night, I was surprised that Steve wasn't there. A lead agent called his apartment, but no one panicked because we figured he'd overslept and was on his way in.

But as time went by, we became increasingly concerned. It wasn't like Steve to disappear without an explanation. I remember huddling with Kenny near the break room, wondering what happened. The premonition of disaster was beginning to tighten its grip.

A short time later, as we began to work on one of the planes, I was called to the main office and told to meet with the night supervisor. Walking into his office, I knew something was terribly wrong. He was pale and would not, or perhaps, could not, look me in the eye, as he calmly explained receiving a call from El Camino Hospital in Mountain View, a town located about ten minutes from where we played ball that same morning. I followed and internalized bits and pieces of what he was saying: There had been a terrible car accident just moments after we left the park…Steve had been thrown from the car…he landed in the brush off the highway…he was critically injured…he was on life support…the Highway Patrol and hospital were trying to contact his family in Boston…it doesn't look good…I'm very sorry, I know you were good friends…I am going to gather the crew and let them know.

I nodded and, without asking for permission, immediately left for the hospital. As I emerged from the office, several employees called out, "Hey, what is up with Steve?" I pretended not to hear, and managed to avoid eye contact.

After leaving the airport, I remember pulling my car off to a side road and bursting into tears. All the partying and recklessness had finally caught up to us. The frightening premonition I had after meeting Agent Dave just weeks ago had come true, and I was completely devastated. To the core of my being, I felt responsible for Steve's accident. That was *my* marijuana and *my* cocaine; it was *my* idea to pick up an additional six pack of beer. There was no denying my responsibility for what happened.

I was the one who always had to push everyone's limits. The last few years had been my personal crusade of rebellion, and now, it had all led to this.

I felt terribly guilty. Everything that Steve did that morning, I had done just as well, maybe even more. How was it that I came home safely and he didn't? I was the one who lacked good judgment and common sense—Steve was the mellow one, the calm, smiling, practical joker who took everything in stride. I was the one with the permanent chip on his shoulder, always looking for an argument or fight, usually against a perceived, but non-existent enemy. Yet, he was in hospital with life-threatening injuries, while I walked around unmarked...at least on the outside.

With the hospital in sight, I actually considered praying. It had been such a long time since I'd sat in the Lord's presence. The journey away from church had been lonely and, deep down, there was always a part of me that wanted to make my way back.

But I remember thinking it might be presumptuous to offer a prayer, especially in light of my behavior the past several years. After all, I relished and celebrated every chance to spit in the face of all I had been taught to believe as a child, and gleefully violated every moral belief and principal I was ever taught. I thought I had pretty well burned my bridges to Church and Faith.

I felt akin to the Prodigal Son in Luke's Gospel, the young man who turned on his family and spent all he had on women and good times, only to return when he had nothing left. I was cut from the same cloth; remarkably self-centered, out for myself, and damn the consequences. There was simply no denying the conscious choices I had made, and now a dear friend lay dying, and I was part of the tragedy.

Pulling up to the bright lights of the hospital parking lot, I couldn't look at myself in the mirror. I didn't feel worthy to pray, so I parked the car and walked through the doors of the Emergency Room alone and in silence.

Once inside, I was directed to the Intensive Care Unit, where I sat and began a long vigil of waiting. In time, a nurse stopped by and let me know that the hospital had made contact with Steve's parents, and they were coming out on the first available flight. I spent the night crying and dozing on and off, and didn't get the chance to see Steve.

The following morning, as word spread about the tragedy, my airline pals began showing up at the hospital. Kenny and I, the last to see Steve alive, were speechless and numb with shock. We had connected with Steve from the moment we'd met him, and were consumed with grief. No doubt, some of the grief was for ourselves and feeling responsible for our behavior that day. We stared vacantly at each other as memories of ball games, beers, and laughs flooded our thoughts. We didn't know what to say; starting a conversation meant having to confront what happened, and our role in it. Instead, we sat quietly, occasionally looking at each other with an encouraging nod of the head, too scared to speak.

Several times I considered calling Mom, but I kept putting it off. I wanted to wait until I had something, anything, positive to offer. I knew she would be devastated for Steve and his family, and painfully disappointed in me. Mom had spoken with me on an almost daily basis, and I simply wouldn't listen. I just had to see my rebellion through on my own terms. I never considered that such recklessness could lead to such darkness.

I think a mom knows the voices of her children, whether they are young, or struggling for adulthood; so when I finally did call, Mom instinctively sensed something was very wrong. I believe she knew it before I uttered a word.

When I explained what happened, she promised prayers for Steve and his parents, and gently suggested that I come home for some rest. I very much wanted to come home…in more ways than one.

A few hours later, without hearing any real news on Steve's condition, I left the hospital and drove home. Mom had coffee ready and held me like a child as I cried for Steve and everyone who was grieving for him. I remember looking up through a teary, swollen face and apologizing to her for my past behavior. She just held me closer and whispered, "I have been worried about you."

I sat at the kitchen table where she always insisted we meet to talk when Maureen, Johnny, and I came home from school as youngsters. I explained how everything about the previous day had seemed so innocent—we were just out to play some ball, have lunch over a few beers, and come home to rest before going to work.

Mom looked at me and shook her head. "You have been running from something ever since we lost Dad, and I have been shocked at your anger. We're all hurting, and we always will, but your anger and attitude the past few years has really worried me. I've never seen you like this. Why don't you tell me what is going on?"

I peered over the top of the cup and mumbled something about "being fine."

Then Mom said, "Why don't you get some sleep. If someone calls, I'll wake you right away. Better yet, why don't you take this time to pray for Steve and his family? You might want to offer a prayer for yourself as well; pray that God will help with all that is going on."

"Pray that God will help? I think we might be past that, Mom," I replied.

"No one is ever past that," she said. "Ever."

And that did it.

The dam burst wide open and a river of venom poured out. It had been building steadily for over a year, and now it exploded from a very deep place within me. "BULLSHIT, MOM, THIS IS SUCH TOTAL BULLSHIT." I'm ashamed of how my language shocked her, but I continued, "Why, Mom? I mean I just don't understand. Why aren't you angry at this God of yours? C'mon, you know, you just have to know that He walked away from Dad, and I'm afraid He will do the same thing to Steve. I want to trust Him, I really do, but I'm kinda afraid He might bail out on us again. After all, that seems to be His history."

At which point, Mom rose up to her full five feet four inch stature and said, "Joseph (it was never a good sign when Mom called me Joseph), you just stop right there." Thirty years later, her words are still ringing in my ears. She explained that while she had no idea why Dad died so suddenly and tragically, there was no doubt in her mind that God was with him—and us—every step of the way. In a plainspoken, direct, manner she assured me that God would also be there when we were all reunited one day in Heaven. Then she paused a moment to let her words sink in, and promptly dropped the haymaker: "Joseph, to me, it seems very immature that you only believe when things are going your way. Real faith means knowing God's love, even when we don't understand it. Only a child walks away when life is difficult. You are not a child, so wake up."

I believe that was the first and only time in my entire life when I have been absolutely speechless.

When Mom finished, I went to the room I grew up in and thought seriously about what she said, and how she said it. I was deeply touched by her words, which came directly from her heart and soul. For me, it was truly, *The Dark Night of The Soul*. Like the great Spanish mystic, John of the Cross, it was time to delve into the darkness and see what it looked like. It was time to stop running and take a good hard look at what I had become. It was also time to see if there was a chance of emerging from this disaster with my soul intact. I felt I had practically given it away throughout the previous year's rebellion. The result was that the core of my being felt empty, as if all the beers and coke had eaten it alive.

Sitting in the quiet of my old bedroom, I focused on the word *Faith*. Just what is it? As a child, faith meant security; it meant that God was with me. However, it also meant that God was in tune with my plan. It was like entering into a bargain with God. I would endure weekend Masses and, in return, God would make sure things went my way. When they didn't go my way...well, I turned my back and walked away.

I remembered how the Sisters from my elementary school days always said that God would always answer our prayers if we asked with a pure heart, but we had to trust in His wisdom. It occurred to me that I'd accepted the former, but had looked past the latter. I accepted that God could answer my prayers, but I neglected to acknowledge that—either way—I needed to trust in His wisdom. As Mom said, "Real faith means believing even when things don't go my way."

It slowly dawned on me that my sense of faith was completely wrapped up within my own sense of *entitlement*. It was more than a little difficult to admit that my faith had never really matured. It was still the faith of a spoiled child.

Spiritually, I hadn't really grown past second or third grade, and the faith I professed in my early twenties was the same as what I'd believed the day of my First Holy Communion, when I was seven.

With such a fragile base, it's no wonder I lost my faith the first time it was tested as an adult. I mean, how can you test an adult who thinks and believes like a child? For me to have lost my faith so quickly after Dad's death meant that the foundation was remarkably weak to begin with. Throughout the Gospels, Jesus implored his disciples to build their faith on rock. Unfortunately, mine was built on soft sand that easily gave way.

I wouldn't go so far as to call the moment an epiphany, but I did acknowledge that Mom was right, and my relationship with the Lord was painfully immature. No wonder I'd never had the feeling of safety or the inner peace I craved. All the beers, marijuana, and cocaine didn't help, either. They certainly did open some unexpected doors of outrageous fun, but in the end, they only led to disaster. They were temporary and momentarily took the edge of life, but they were certainly not a long term solution.

I began to feel that I was *finally* making some progress; enough, at least, to begin looking at the quality of my faith and begin taking a long, hard look at the effect of my using. In all honesty, I don't think I was anywhere close to completely giving it up and walking away...but it was a start.

At least I had a real sense that the game was up because the cost was too high, and it was, at last, time to be honest and humble with what had become of my life. I felt the Lord's presence in a new and very reassuring way. It was as if He was gently whispering through the darkness. *"OK, Joe, come home to me. Come off that weary road and rest within my healing love."*

It was beautifully soothing.

For the first time since my argument with God in the meditation room outside Dad's hospital room, I didn't feel alone and lost. Sure, his death would forever haunt me, but it's not the same as blaming God for it. It is not the same as accusing God of abandoning us.

For the first time, I felt that maybe there was an alternative view to my spiritual frustration and rage. Maybe Jesus, who also knew suffering and loss, could actually walk with me through this or any other pain in my life. Fighting Him simply didn't work, and it only led to increased misery. So maybe the key was to humbly ask His forgiveness and seek a healing reconciliation. I figured at this point, *anything* was better than walking around in a perpetual state of anger and bitterness, half out of my mind on drugs and alcohol.

As the long night continued, I had a sense that the beaten and battered Jesus, the Jesus who knew heartache, betrayal, and suffering, would understand where I had been and where I hoped to go. I began to feel that He truly understood having been there Himself. Maybe the key was simply to ask Him to join me on the journey…no promises, no agendas, no demands…just a simple promise to walk with me. I kneeled at the side of the bed and humbly asking Jesus of The Cross to join me on this new journey.

8
The Death of Steve Olsen

The next morning, I returned to El Camino Hospital and met Steve's parents, who had just arrived from Boston. I was nervous about meeting Gerald and Ruth Olsen, and had prepared myself for the worst while driving to the hospital. I expected Steve's parents to take at least some of their hurt out on me. I imagined Mr. Olsen confronting me, "So, you're Joe, the smart ass who always had to push it. Now look what you've done."

I was dreading it, but fully expecting it at the same time. I remember parking my car and whispering, "Jesus, I really need you. I am sorry for all I did to help instigate this disaster, and I am sorry for hurting You in the last year for not being the man I was raised to be, but I ask that You please walk with me. I'll take what I have coming because I deserve it, but I'll feel better, and stronger if I know You are by my side." With that I walked to the ICU room to meet Steve's parents.

When I arrived at Steve's room, his parents came out and met me in the hall. Mr. Olsen gently shook my hand and asked if I was all right, while Mrs. Olsen hugged me and gave me a kiss on my cheek. I was moved to tears. They just poured out and wouldn't stop. I was prepared for a bruising lecture, but from the very beginning, it was clear that neither were interested in casting judgment. There would be plenty of time to discuss the harsh lessons as time moved along.

Mr. Olsen took my arm and gently walked me to Steve's bedside. He looked frightening with a breathing tube and IV's inserted throughout his body. Just mere hours ago he had been such an amazing athlete, and now he looked so beaten and battered. It was a shock.

A nurse came over and put her arm around me and said, "Your friend doesn't feel anything."

I know she meant well and was just trying to help, but I disagreed with her assessment. I believed Steve felt *everything.* I thought he could feel and sense everything and everyone who was there praying for him.

His California buddies (his Dad's words for us) gathered in the waiting room and quietly prayed. Mr. Olsen came out from time to time and gave us updates, but Mrs. Olsen never left her son's side. We marked time by sharing a few stories with Mr. Olsen about Steve's life in California. We spoke of how much we cared for him and how his sense of humor was completely over the top. Through a steady stream of tears, we shared our profound regrets over what happened. No one shied away from the truth. We loved him and were consumed with heartache over the tragedy.

Steve remained in a coma for a week. During that time, I kept a silent vigil every day. I would use the time to reflect on where I'd been. Sometimes I would simply remain silent and feel the Lord's presence. It wasn't a dramatic spiritual transition; it was very subtle, but real. Kenny, an airline employee who was equally close to Steve, was my constant companion. Occasionally, we would break the tension by breaking into laughter at some of our fond memories, but for the most part we sat in silence.

I had always respected Kenny, though a quick look at us and one might think we had nothing in common: I, the white Catholic, raised in Catholic schools, and Kenny, an African-American Baptist, educated in public schools. But the truth is, we had everything in common. We were both brought up in close, tight-knit, faith-filled families; we had parents with strong community values; and we shared a devotion to sports, which we played and watched as often as possible. He had been in our home, and I had been in his. We were close yet, with all that as history, the enormity of the accident rendered us both speechless.

Throughout the long days of vigil and reflection, we noticed a priest walking through the halls stopping at various rooms. One afternoon, he emerged from Steve's room with Mr. Olsen at his side, locked in conversation. When they returned we could tell that Mr. Olsen had been crying, but the instant he saw us sitting quietly in the waiting room, he straightened up, composed himself, and walked toward us, with the priest not far behind.

The priest impressed me with his generosity and his time. He seemed completely relaxed around our motley crew of scared young men and women, and had a nice way of looking you in the eye and being present to the situation without saying anything trite or superficial. When he told us, "I offered Mass for all of you this morning, and you are very much in my prayers," we knew he meant it.

Mr. Olsen sat down and told Kenny and I that Steve wasn't going to make it. He had to say it a second time because his words didn't connect with either of us. "Fellas, Steve's injuries are too severe, and we have to let him go."

We allowed the horror of his words to sink in, and then joined the priest in a prayer. I don't know about Kenny, but for me, the prayer was more a plea than an actual prayer. I asked the broken and battered Jesus of the Cross to be with my friend and continue loving him. I, again, asked for forgiveness for my actions the day of the accident, and forgive me for the life choices I'd made the year leading up to the tragedy.

The following morning was Easter Sunday, April, 1980.

My friend, Steve, died peacefully with his parents at his bedside. I have no doubt that God welcomed him to eternal rest and peace with love. I also know that the loss of Steve Olsen and the horrible manner in which he died have had a lifelong effect on me. I believe his death was the event that pushed me toward another path and back on the original road I'd started as a youngster.

I am a priest today because of what happened to Steve that April morning. It was the tragic event that forced me to reconsider how I was living and humbly seek another way. There is no doubt in my mind that Steve spiritually interceded on my behalf and helped turn my life around. I believe that at home and at rest in the peace of God Steve watched out for me and all the old airport gang. His presence, like my dad's, was spiritual but, nonetheless, real.

Shortly after his passing, Steve's body was gently placed in the belly of an airplane for the long trip home to Boston. The lead agent allowed Steve's friends to enter the cargo area in the belly of the plane for a few moments of prayer. There were choked tears of grief, but no one said anything. Holding hands, we knelt by the casket and offered words from the silence of our hearts. Kenny and I were the last to leave, and we hugged each other and promised Steve that we would fly to Boston and attend his funeral Mass.

Life at the airline was never the same again. It seemed like a bridge had been crossed, and there was no going back. The never-ending parties, the recklessness, the drug and alcohol abuse—all of it had led to tragedy. Even the travel ceased being fun. In fact, after flying home from Steve's funeral, I never flew again. My flying and partying days were over.

I was consumed with guilt. For months, even years, I saw Steve's face everywhere. I would wake up seeing his parents at the hospital and his brother and sisters at the funeral Mass. It haunted me. I suppose there was an element of survivor guilt. Kenny and I knew that what happened to Steve could easily have happened to us. But our feelings went deeper; we knew that we would forever share in the tragedy of Steve's death. It would be a huge burden to carry for the rest of our lives.

There is a story the French philosopher and novelist, Albert Camus, once told about a young man who, while sitting on the bank of the River Seine near Paris, watched a woman slip off the embankment and fall into the water. The man watched as she slowly submerged beneath the water while fighting for her life. Several times he started to get up to help, but he always fell back and watched passively. Eventually, despite a courageous struggle, the woman slipped deep into the water and drowned. His failure to act, his failure to do the right thing haunted him for the rest of his life, to the point where he considered taking his own life. Many years later, the now elderly man returned to bank of the river and started to walk into the water. It reached his knees, then his waist, then his neck. Then he stopped and looked up the heavens and shouted, "Oh woman, come down into these waters, that I may reach out and save both of us."

That is how I feel about Steve to this day. I wish we hadn't been drinking and driving that day, and I wish I could go back in time and keep him out of that car. I wish we hadn't gone out for beers, and I wish I hadn't brought extra beer and drugs with me. *I wish, I wish, I wish.* I wish I could have saved him. But I have no doubt that safe and at peace in his home with God in Heaven, my friend, Steve, reached out and helped save me.

Postscript: Steve's life and death not only affected and changed the course of my life, but it also impacted the direction of Kenny's as well. Today, Kenny serves as a leader in the Baptist community in Atlanta, Georgia, where he offers counsel to youngsters, and high risk youth. God bless you, Kenny.

Postscript: In my research for this book, I spoke at length with members of Steve's family. Almost thirty years after his death, I recently learned that Mr. and Mrs. Olsen gave permission for Steve's organs to be harvested for transplant. And so it was, that through Steve and the generosity of his family, someone else received the gift and blessing of new life. As one who has received a heart transplant, I cannot begin to express my prayerful gratitude to the Olsen family for their decision at a time of terrible loss. My love and prayers are with them forever.

The Second Gift:
Sobriety and Ordination as a Priest

9

A Rough Road

I think if you're going to write a memoir it has to be honest. I don't think it would be fair to slick it up so it has a nice, neat, happy, Disney feel to it. I think it has to be real, warts and all. Reader beware: Here come the ugly warts.

My journey to sobriety and ordination as a Catholic priest was not smooth.

Not by a long shot.

A part of me that wants to say that after Steve's death, I never went near drugs or alcohol ever again. It might make for a nice story and a beautiful tribute to Steve, but it would be a lie. I was much more careful, but I still drank and used; perhaps not as often, but it was still part of my life. It seemed like I always needed something extra in my life for balance and excitement.

I did make some lifestyle changes following Steve's death, but looking back, I realize that it was mostly superficial. There wasn't a lot of introspection involved, but there was a certain desire to move past the days of old when recklessness defined my every thought and action. I did my level best to keep my drinking and using under control and hidden from the rest of the world. I stopped stealing liquor off planes and even began the long, slow, rehabilitation of my reputation at work. I stopped attending airline social gatherings and even refrained from joining members of the work crew for the occasional   beer after work. I went underground and tried to keep my drinking a private affair.

But that didn't stop me from pulling into a liquor store or convenience market and picking up a few beers to savor on the way home. I tried to be as covert as possible, and disciplined myself to avoid drinks at social functions. My pals *almost* believed I had walked away from the life. I became quite the sneak at hiding my drinking and pot smoking from others. I even secured another dealer who didn't work at the airport and had no connection to my friends.

However, with time, I slowly slipped back into the old ways. It was nowhere near as reckless as past years, but I picked my spots and managed to keep myself in control. At least, I convinced myself I had it in control. Sadly, I still felt I needed it. When life became stressed, I still felt that pull to reach back for a drink or relax at the end of a pipe. Deep down I didn't want to go back, but the pull was powerful. It seemed the more I "white knuckled" and fought it, the stronger it became. While it was much more low-key, it was still there.

10

Who is Thomas Merton, and How Did He Encourage my Vocation to the Priesthood?

For my twenty-first birthday, one of my uncles gave me a book, *The Seven Story Mountain*, the autobiography of Thomas Merton. I thanked him for the book and tossed it on the shelf in my room, where it sat for the next six months.

One afternoon, I picked it up, wiped away the dust, and for all practical purposes I never put it down. Thirty years later, I still read sections from time to time. Thomas Merton was from a different time and generation, and he touched a nerve in me that remains alive to this day. His life was influential in reclaiming my interest to become a Catholic priest. That it was inspired by a monk who lived in a monastery for twenty-seven years before dying in 1969, is a tribute to his brilliant writing and insightful commentaries.

The title refers to the mountain of purgatory in Dante's *Divine Comedy*, and covers Merton's days of being orphaned as a young man and wandering throughout Europe and America in search of himself. While a brilliant student, he was rudderless. He felt alone and was constantly searching for a "center" in his life to give him the peace he longed for. I felt connected to his journey from the first page.

Eventually, after years of drinking and loneliness, he finds what he is looking for at the Abbey of Gethsemane, a Trappist Monastery in Kentucky. Besides his autobiography, he kept journals that spoke of his past and his ongoing need for contemplative prayer and solitude. Eventually, Thomas sought permission from the Abbott to live outside the monastery grounds as a hermit.

I became a Merton addict. I just couldn't get enough of this brilliant and unusual man who walked away from a teaching and writing job at Columbia University to live in a quiet monastery in the heart of Kentucky.

As I read of his exploits and spiritual journey, I found myself returning to my original thoughts of priesthood. The attraction of Merton was the fact that he had lived a complicated life, and his story was not a smooth road to the monastery. There were plenty of bumps and bruises along the way, and he had his share of mistakes and regrets. At the risk of hubris, I thought we actually had something in common—neither of us were saints and neither followed a simple path to priesthood.

I found myself reflecting on a key point that Thomas referred to several times in his various journals: The epic battle (we all face) between our "True Self" and our "False Self." The latter is the way we want others to see us; it's the facade we put up for the world. For me, the "False Self" was all things related to drinking and using. Under the influence, I often felt strong and confident, the life of the party; except it was a mere show. It was a fraudulent production of something that wasn't real. It was my "False Self."

The "True Self" is the way God sees us. It is who we really are as children of God, as children of light and hope. The spiritual journey of Thomas Merton was all about claiming and reclaiming his "True Self." For me, my "True Self" is the man who is truly free; free to live, love, and serve with happiness and joy. I can gracefully accept me for who I really am without putting on false airs to please others.

I remembered my wild days at the airport when I was like a chameleon—I would literally change personas and alter my personality depending on the mix of drugs I was using. Quite the opposite of being free, I was a slave to my own self destructive need to use and drink, even if it was just for a quick temporary high.

Like Thomas, I wanted to reclaim my "True Self," honestly believing that such a pursuit would lead me to applying to the seminary. My life had been such a spiritual roller coaster. I was raised happily close to the church, but had fallen away from all spiritual matters and concerns, only to survive and — at least attempt — to find my way back to the beginning. There was a certain circular element to it, and now I hoped to revisit and walk the journey as it first began.

I spent months in prayer wondering if my past behavior would get in the way of a vocation. I seriously doubted if there were seminarians who drank, used, stole, and had a record of gleefully walking away from the Church quite like I did. There was a big part of me that could see the Vocation Director laughing me out of the building once he got a clear sense of my history. Still, I felt God was using me in some way, maybe to simply use what I learned to teach others to keep them from making the same mistakes. In the end, I made peace with the idea of beginning the application process. If the seminary rejected me, I would simply and respectfully honor it as God's will.

One afternoon, I sat at the same kitchen table with Mom where we had our little chat about faith on the eve of Steve's death. It had been several years since his passing, and I had rejoined Mom at Mass and a variety of church events. So much of my life had changed since the tragedy, and our kitchen table seemed like the perfect location to discuss a completely new direction.

"I know I've put you through a lot, Mom, and you stayed with me through some very dark days. Now, at last, I'm ready to do what I wanted as a much younger man. I want to serve God and others as a priest, and think I might have a message that can help others. I honestly don't know if they will accept me, but I would like to apply…and I wanted you to be the first to know."

Mom's response was just what I expected, "That you are at peace is the most important thing to me — where you find it is up to you. I'm very happy for you, and deep down, I'm not all that surprised."

It was the kind of measured reaction I expected from Mom; ever true to form, her only interest was that Maureen, Johnny, and I would find happiness and peace in our journey through life.

Suffice it to say that my sister's reaction was somewhat different. "What?" she exclaimed, "are you serious? OK, what is *really* going on? Look, I know you were shaken by the investigation, and I totally understand your emotions about Steve's death, but c'mon, you can't honestly believe you're going to find peace and happiness there."

I think Maureen saw life in the seminary as a scene from a medieval monastery, where her older brother was locked in a closet copying manuscripts for the rest of his life. Many years later, with the advantage of hindsight, I asked her if she cared to illuminate her initial reaction. Maureen replied, "I always saw you as married with a family, and I wondered if you were running away from something. I guess my vision of life for you was very different from your own—I thought you would choose a more *normal* path."

Turns out, my sister wasn't the only one who had such feelings. I think Maureen's reaction, in light of my recent history, was an accurate portrait of how my extended family and friends felt about my application to the seminary. While no one was going to lock and bar the doors and windows, they seriously questioned my motivation. Most felt that it was a psychological reaction to the tragic events of the past years. I don't think anyone thought my journey to the seminary would last very long.

My younger brother, John, was characteristically upbeat. "Look, I'd just like to see you happy. If this is what you want to do with your life, I'll back you all the way."

While surprised, neither my brother nor sister tried to talk me out of the decision. No doubt, they had their concerns and misgivings, but in the end, they were both willing to offer unconditional love and support.

11

Application to College Seminary

In the days leading up to my formal interview, I fought a real internal battle with myself. I was at peace, but I just didn't see any way the Archdiocese of San Francisco would ever accept me as a seminarian. In fact, I almost walked away from the initial interview but decided that for once in my life I would actually face my fears and doubts and see it through.

Walking up the steps to the Chancery Office, I was convinced that once the appropriate authorities got wind of my past history, they would turn their backs and flee in the opposite direction. My college background was limited to two years of study, and my experience in the parish was confined to my high school days of youth ministry; hardly a glowing resume of spiritual commitment. I had also recently lost a dear friend and was about to freely admit to lying, stealing, and using in the final years before applying. I was determined that, if nothing else, I would be honest throughout the interview. I didn't want to (possibly) start a new path in life by playing a game of deception and loading my answers with outright lies and half-truths. My interview might be raw and emotional, but at least it would be honest. If the Catholic Church chose to accept my application, they would know exactly who and what they were getting. Still, deep down, I couldn't shake the nagging feeling that this might be the shortest interview of my life.

Fr. Bruce Dreier was the Vocation Director for the Archdiocese of San Francisco. He would, ultimately, be responsible for recommending or rejecting my application. Additionally, he would be the priest who would speak directly to the Archbishop as to my "readiness" for entry into the college seminary.

He was a large man whose size was almost betrayed by his soft, gentle voice. He quickly shared that he hadn't applied to seminary until his college days were over and he had "lived a little."

I nodded, "I'm sure glad to hear you say that, Father, because I have lived a little."

With that I launched into my history, warts, regrets, and everything in between. When I finished, Fr. Bruce thanked me for my honesty and proceeded with several more questions. To my surprise he didn't boot me out the door on the spot. In fact, he seemed genuinely grateful at my honesty, and was more than willing to continue the discussion. For the first time since receiving the appointment to meet, I actually relaxed.

It felt good sharing the truth of my life, regardless of the outcome. When your life is wrapped around drinking and using, the truth is the one thing you really fear. I'd told so many lies during my airline days that I didn't even know what the truth was. There were times I was so mixed up I honestly didn't even know what I'd said and to whom I had said it. I was constantly back-checking my "facts" just to keep the various stories straight. It was an incredible waste of time and energy, but under the influence, I would speak the first thought that entered my clouded mind. There just wasn't a whole hell of a lot of integrity involved in any of my relationships.

Fr. Bruce proved to be an adroit listener and intuitive questioner. Rather than immediately launch into the "why's" and "how's" I dug myself such a hole, he refocused the conversation and asked, "Joe, what is it about Jesus that inspires you to leave the past behind and follow him?"

I remember repeating the words and thoughts from my childhood; to me, Jesus was the ultimate man of healing and peace. I had always been deeply touched by His humility. He certainly had the chance to become a King as our world understands it, but He consciously chose to live as a servant to the poorest of the poor. I admired that He defended those who could not always defend themselves.

I told Fr. Bruce about a man I worked for at the airline. He was a thoroughly decent guy and great to work for because I respected his leadership style. He'd come out years ago as a gay man and was subsequently diagnosed with the AIDS virus. He ended up leaving work to spend his final days at home. None of us, including me, ever went to visit...or call...or write...and I was ashamed because he was always very nice and respectful to me, even when I did nothing but cause trouble. He actually died weeks before I even knew it.

I felt that Jesus would have been at his door at the first sign of trouble. He would have cared for the poor man and offered hope throughout his struggle. I felt Jesus was the ONE to break down walls and barriers of ignorance and prejudice.

I also believed that this same Jesus had walked with me through some very dark times, and I wanted to help people as He had helped me. I simply wanted to be His minister—not for any fancy title or distinguished clerical uniform, but to give back what I had received. I concluded by saying, "The honest truth is maybe I will wash out of your seminary for a host of reasons, but I really feel called to give it a chance. I feel I have been given the gift of reclaiming my faith for a reason and I want to share it as a dedicated priest."

Fr. Dreier offered an approving smile and said he would be in touch soon. As is standard practice, he set up an interview with the Archdiocesan counselor and asked that I take an academic placement test as well.

It was several months later when I received a letter from Archbishop John R. Quinn saying that I had been accepted into the college seminary. I would study philosophy and undergo a two year formation program before applying to the major seminary. All said, I would be on a seven year track to ordination.

God help us all.

12
Saying Goodbye to the Airline

I think it is safe to say that no one, and I mean *no one*, could believe the news that one of our employees was leaving the airline to enter a Catholic seminary. When the crew learned that someone was me, well, the shock was deafening. No one could believe it. Part of it was my fault. In the long year of prayer and discernment, I hadn't spoken to anyone about my interest. Also, for several years, I had zealously nurtured a reputation as a self-professed hell raiser. No one pushed the limits of common sense and appropriate behavior quite like I did, and no one was more disrespectful of rules and obligations than I. So when the crew heard the word, they didn't know whether to laugh or just shake their heads in disbelief.

Truthfully, I'd been too embarrassed to even bring it up. I was the anarchist of the group who often offended the older employees with caustic remarks about all things related to God and Faith. I believed in nothing and no one. I lived for fun. Period. So who could blame the old gang for laughing off the notion that I might enter a Catholic seminary? They must have thought, "How could Joe possibly have slipped through the admissions process? Don't they screen people? Lord, what will happen to our Church?"

While it was true that I had really pulled back from all the parties and travel since Steve's death, leaving the airline business to enter a Catholic seminary was simply beyond comprehension to my old pals. I understood. For most of my friends, priests were straight out of *Going my Way* or *Bells of St. Mary's*, with Bing Crosby as the wise, paternal, pastor with impeccable insight and knowledge of the human condition. I didn't exactly fit the mold. The image of the paternal "Bing" was miles apart from how they knew me.

Having said that, the work crew was painfully polite about my new venture, and they even managed not to laugh while I was in the room. But privately, the general sentiment was that once I got a better look at the seminary, and more importantly, once the seminary got a better look at *me*, I would soon be back where I belonged, traveling all over the country and raising mischief throughout the airport.

The traditional "Goodbye" party offered to employees who were moving to other cities or jobs was quietly dispensed for my leaving. I'm positive most of the lead agents were delighted to be rid of me, no doubt an answer their prayer, and the crew was simply too stunned to move on anything.

They did, however, start the Official Airline Seminary Pool. For a mere ten dollars, you could purchase a block that included the date and time I would be unceremoniously booted from the seminary. I hadn't begun to pack, but already there was a line waiting to wager on a sure thing.

13

St. Joseph's College Seminary

I was so nervous on the day I entered St. Josephs' College Seminary that I stopped at a pub less than ten miles away from the seminary grounds and downed half a pitcher of beer, thinking it might take the edge off before beginning a new life.

The morning began with the family gathered at Mom's house for an enormous breakfast. Mom and Maureen were in tears as I packed up the car, but Johnny kept a stiff upper lip while reminding me if I wasn't happy, I could always come home.

I drove off unsteadily and, less than a mile from home, made up my mind to stop for a cold one when I was near the seminary, and pick up a six pack of beer, which I would hide for safe keeping in the trunk of my car.

Nice way to start a new phase of life.

The fact that I was starting anew while still clinging to the old ways of the past never registered; or, if it did, I chose to ignore it. I was in the seminary, far from everything and everyone else from my recent past, and that's all that mattered. I wanted solitude and time to reflect on what happened the last few years. I wanted to pull back and take a good look at myself, and the seminary offered the chance to do so. Ultimately, I would have seven years to consider priesthood, so I wasn't rushing into anything. The thought of a tall draft beer seemed like a good way to ease into the process.

St. Joseph's College Seminary was a two-year program based on the model of discernment; that is, I would have time to prayerfully consider my vocation while carrying a full academic schedule of classes. In turn, the faculty and staff would have two years to observe me. After two years, they would vote whether I was ready to move on to St. Patrick's Seminary for the final years of formation.

In many ways, the only difference between my last year at the airline and my first year in the college seminary was I was living in the hills, sixty miles south of the airport. The same issues followed me right through the main doors of St. Joseph's. Once the novelty of entering the seminary wore off, I basically went straight back into the same lifestyle I had at the airport. The names were different, but the scam was just the same. In fact, the only real change was that I'd learned to become more careful, more deceitful in finding ways to drink and use. My activities were covert, and I avoided the spotlight. I learned to hide in the shadows.

Often when people think of life in a college seminary, they think of a monastery, complete with a strict closed-door policy where the seminarians live like cloistered monks in an abbey. They see people walking around in silence muttering prayers under their breath.

That wasn't the case at St. Joseph's. For the most part we were free to come and go as we pleased. Of course, we were responsible for being on time and attentive at all our classes and formational seminars, but we had plenty of free time. We were expected to be at morning and evening prayer and daily mass, but there were still opportunities to cultivate relationships and go out on the town. The weekends, although filled with homework and study for endless exams, were still basically ours to do with as we pleased.

The atmosphere was a far cry from past times when seminarians lived in a locked-down atmosphere. In those days, they had to apply for permission to leave the seminary anytime during the week. They only met with people "outside the gates" on official Visiting Days, which occurred every few months. By contrast, I drove home several weekends each month for some home cooking and checked in with old friends.

In the college seminary, there were a few young seminarians in their late teens, and an equally few in their late fifties, but the vast majority of the students were in their mid-twenties or early thirties. Almost all had completed college and arrived with B.A. degrees in a wide variety of subjects. I was one of the very few without a college degree so, in terms of academics, I was really starting from ground zero.

It didn't take long to formulate a few friendships with seminarians who shared a similar background with me. After a long day of classwork, one of the fellas would drive to a local convenience store and bring a six pack of beer home with him, where we would hide the beer in the closest and share them during a "study session" later in the evening. There was no explicit rule against consuming alcohol—*in moderation*—but, as usual, I walked a fine line thinking I had it under control, while still drinking almost every day to take the edge off.

It didn't affect my studies, and I was very careful to pick my spots. For example, I *never* drank at faculty/seminarian social gatherings. I would walk around nursing a mineral water, and later, disappear to my room to quickly down a beer or quick shot of Jack. I would follow it up with a gulp of mouth wash, and then quietly return to the social. I began to cultivate a double life: dutiful seminarian by day, serious drinker every other chance I got.

I was doing the same thing in a Catholic seminary that I did while working for a major airline. Sure, my behavior was less reckless and, by this time, I knew the importance of keeping a low profile, but I was definitely doing the same things. I mixed in with the community, never said anything controversial, kept my grades up through long hours of study, but basically remained the same, slick, drinker I was in the last year of work at the airport. I was just much more adept at hiding it.

I knew the price of being visible, so I kept a low profile and smiled and laughed when appropriate. They were lessons I learned at the airport the hard way, and I didn't want to make the same mistakes twice.

One day an old airline pal called and offered to come up and visit. After giving him the grand tour and assuring him of my happiness, we shuffled into my room where he unveiled a present from several members of the old gang: a large bottle of Jack Daniels and a healthy bag of marijuana. I thanked him, told him to send my love to the crew, and hid the treasures in my tiny closet.

Because my grades were more than respectable and I never missed a class, Mass, or prayer service, the faculty looked at me as a solid, mature seminarian who was dedicated to his studies and mixed well in the community. I was playing yet another scam with a different group of people. I wanted to live in both worlds by doing well in seminary while still holding on to the ways of the past.

I became quite accomplished at playing the game. While shopping for bottled water, I would sneak a few miniature bottles of whiskey—the same ones I used to steal from incoming flights—into the shopping bag and walk right past faculty members sitting and chatting in the front parlor.

Same game; different place.

Thirty years later, I am ashamed that I took advantage of their trust and goodness.

By now, it was pretty obvious I couldn't find happiness without a few beers or toke of marijuana in my system. Even in the relatively structured environment of a Catholic seminary, I still clung to the notion that I could keep my drinking and using under control. The sad truth is whether cleaning airplanes, loading baggage, or studying to be a Catholic priest, I couldn't imagine life without it. It was part of me, and behind *every* decision I made.

Eventually, (of course) I started bringing more than one six pack to my room. I would hide the extra one in my closet or desk drawer. If I drank too much, I would lock the door, put on headphones, and slip off to sleep. I kept a real low profile in the hope that none of the seminarians would know I was missing.

Looking back, I'm amazed how easy it was to slip into the ways of the past. Basically, during that first year at St. Joseph's, I cultivated a double life which allowed me to study and prepare for classes, while still nurturing my love for beer and marijuana. I studied hard, trying to grasp complex philosophical presentations, but would calmly disappear from time to time to hit various bars and pubs a short distance away from the seminary grounds. When I came home,

I would carefully watch that no one was hanging out in front of the building, then walk directly to my room on the fourth floor. I didn't want to call any unnecessary attention to myself. If someone saw me I would always look directly at them and wave with a big smile as if I had nothing to hide.

But I was hiding from everything and everyone. I wish I had realized that having to hide is often the first indication that a problem exists.

The next morning, I would walk purposefully into the chapel for prayer and respectfully take my seat as if nothing happened the previous evening. Regardless how hung over I often felt, I never missed a beat. I felt that as long as my attendance was perfect, everything must be all right.

In spite of my closet drinking and using, I enjoyed the communal life at St. Joseph's. My problem was I wanted everything. I wanted to have a good spiritual life, but still drank like a fish. I wanted to have the integrity of a seminarian, but still hid in my room with a pipe. I wanted to be honest with the priests and staff, but had to lie to cover myself. It became more and more complicated each day. That is what happens when there is a total lack of integrity about what you're doing.

In time, I became close friends with another seminarian. We were both a little older than many of the students and had lived "out in the world." He had a wonderful sense of humor and kept all of us in good spirits with his ability to tell a good story. He did, however, bring the same issues I brought to the seminary. He was equally good at hiding his desires and needs, but they were as real for him as they were for me. Since we had so much in common, we became close friends, opening up to each other and sharing our stories. We quickly joined ranks in escaping once or twice a week.

Working as a tag team required an innate sense of timing. One of us would watch the driveway while the other went for the car (whoever had the most gas in the tank was the automatic driver). Then we'd meet at the front gate, hop in the car and visit a few pubs in nearby Los Altos or Palo Alto. While it's true the gate was never locked, the faculty kept their eyes wide open for guys heading out too many times during the week. Caution was the order of the day, and the last thing a seminarian wanted to do was call undo attention to himself. Such attention would lead to questions, which would bring the seminary staff into the picture—not a good place to be if you are cultivating a double life.

The last weekend of the fall semester as we prepped for final exams, my friend entered my room and produced a small white baggie with an odd white powder. From experience, I immediately knew it wasn't cocaine, and he quickly explained it was methamphetamine, and it would keep us awake for a few hours of extra study. It also had a nice, euphoric kick that was just the thing to get us through the final weeks.

As I watched him empty some a small amount on my desk, it occurred to me that rather than moving forward, I was actually moving in reverse. If you worked it carefully, and tossed integrity out the window, St. Joseph's could be a lovely place to hide from your demons. In my case, I'd packed them up and brought them with me.

You haven't changed a damn bit, I noted to myself as I watched him cut up the meth. While critiquing myself, I instinctively began rolling a dollar bill to use as a straw to snort the drug. *Hell, you're even worse than before because you're smarter and more devious this time around.*

Although I truly respected the seminary and the priests who ran it, I was making a mockery of it...and a mockery of myself. Deep down, I didn't want to live like this. I really wanted to give St. Joseph's a chance, but I couldn't stop drinking and using.

I remember looking almost sorrowful at my buddy, and finally blurting out, "You know, drugs are like a beautiful woman to me. Even if I know she doesn't care about me, even if I know I'll get dumped and feel hurt, and have regrets, I still want to be around her because I still think I'll eventually be happy with her. Even when I know it's not going to happen, and it will end ugly, I still want to be near her."

"There has to be a certain insanity attached to this," I mused. "We both came here to pursue something sacred and real, and we're doing the same thing that initially made us so miserable and unhappy. We must be nuts. I mean, there is no way this is normal. I'm feeling really guilty about this."

Of course, this self-directed outrage did *not* prevent me from sampling what my friend brought home. I actually did a line (the first time in a long time) and remained awake throughout the night with my good friends Plato and Socrates. In fact, I used the drug several times throughout the week and rarely slept while preparing for my first set of seminary exams.

I developed an amazing ability to separate using from the rest of my orderly life in the seminary. I actually sampled a tiny bit of meth a half hour before one of the exams later in the week. When the professor handed out the blue books for our answers, I was flying. I felt so wired that I filled the whole book and finished early. I don't know how, but I actually received a high mark. Exams complete, I went back to my room and slept on and off for two days during our midterm break.

My ability to compartmentalize was shocking even to me. I worked hard to maintain a solid, dependable, mature presence in the community, while privately violating every rule in the book. Life was a dichotomy between the reality of living as a seminarian and a guy who simply loved to drink and use.

Living a double life is really hard, regardless of what we do for a living. But living a double life as a seminarian is especially brutal because people are putting their faith in you; my family and people from my home parish were sending cards, letters, and occasional food packages, and I was betraying their trust.

My brother and sister, just starting their adult lives, were sending me money so I could go to a movie or have dinner out sometime, and I was using it for beer and marijuana. The more I did it, the more my esteem plummeted, and the more my esteem plummeted, the more I did it.

It was physically and emotionally taxing, and it almost destroyed any sense I had of spirituality. I was constantly ashamed of myself, but I lacked a plan or idea how to get out of the hole I had built for years. It was a very dark and isolated and lonely place.

I remember one afternoon, walking into my tiny room and pausing because it smelled of empty beer cans and bottles. I opened the window and literally scrubbed the room for hours, trying to get rid of the smell in case a professor or faculty priest popped in for quick visit. I didn't know if it the smell was all that bad or if it was my own paranoia, but I was taking no chances. I wrapped all the cans and bottles and tossed them into the outdoor garbage cans. I breathed a sigh of relief and went back to my room, where it still reeked of stale beer.

We were expected to meet each week with our faculty advisor; mine was a rather blunt, direct man named, Fr. Robert Evers. At one of our meetings he looked at me for a long time then noted, "I like you, Joe, I think you're funny as can be and I like your personality. But I've been wondering whether you're here because you are running away from something…or someone. Now, bullshit your Bishop and Vocation Director if you must, but please have a little respect and be honest with me. What is really going on with you? I have a sense you're hiding something. Let me in."

I was stunned. It was one of the very few times anyone had called me on anything. I decided his rather brutal question called for an equally blunt response. "The truth is, Father, sometimes I wonder myself. There are times when I'm alone with the Lord in chapel and I wonder if I'm running *from* something or *to* something. To be honest, I don't know. Maybe I'm running from past mistakes and failures. Maybe I'm running away from the airport where I worked and got into a whole lot of trouble. I'm not sure." I stammered and almost whispered, "I think I'm still getting used to living in a seminary, and maybe some of the old life is still in me."

It was the best I could do, the closest I could get to a confession. No doubt, I was still clinging perilously to several issues from my past. Despite believing that I had everything in

control, there was part of me that could feel it slipping
away…again.

Fr. Evers offered a half smile, but noted, "Good for you, I'm
glad to hear it. This isn't a place to hide. Whatever you brought
with you will stay with you. In fact, it will get worse…you can
count on that."

His words haunted me as I returned to the solitude of my
room, and I knew he was right. But I still kept going. Fr. Evers was
a very smart and experienced priest, and I was concerned he was
on to me. I decided to be extra careful and cease slipping out at
night. I actually liked my life at St. Joseph's. I enjoyed my
classmates and admired and respected the faculty professors. But I
was also worried that some well-intentioned soul would find out
what I was up to.

Several nights after dinner, I would stop by the rooms of
several of the professors and receive clarification regarding the
morning or afternoon lecture. I would usually start by asking if it
was delivered, "in English or Latin?" They were generous with
their time because they wanted us to do well. But there was one
professor who absolutely terrified anyone and everyone who dared
cross a path into his classroom: Fr. David Thayer, St. Joseph's
legendary taskmaster and Chair of the Philosophy Department.

My first impression? The man was an intellectual sadist.

Fr. Thayer had a bombastic voice and an imposing frame. He
had this habit of routinely dropping words and phrases I couldn't
quite decipher. Once, before a midterm exam, we entered his
classroom to find the following words on the blackboard:

"Gentlemen, remember an F+ means defeat with honor."

See what I mean? An intellectual sadist if there ever was one.

At first, I was thoroughly convinced he was, in fact, evil. But as
time went by, I learned that it was all just a front. He cared deeply
about the progress of his students and would go to any length to
help—if he felt we were sincere. He believed it was his role to attack
and break down every preconceived theological notion and
philosophical concept we dared to bring to his classroom, and then

rebuild it from a more mature, inquiring perspective. It took some time, but I came to genuinely admire him as a teacher and as a priest.

He turned out to be quite merciful with grunts like me who entered his classroom with all senses focused on survival; but he was absolutely brutal to the younger guys, especially those who majored in philosophy and had serious hierarchal goals (like Bishop). To those poor lads, he was vicious and unforgiving. He would sarcastically shred every point they made in class, while guys like me would just sit back and watch the show.

Near the end of my second year, I became increasingly frustrated with the study of philosophy. I was looking for answers, and philosophy just seemed to pose endless questions. In fact, every time I understood a particular philosophical belief, Fr. Thayer would turn it around and offer a totally different vision that made even more sense. I usually walked out of his class utterly clueless as to the point he was making.

One day as the process continued, he asked if there were any questions. I couldn't resist raising my hand. "Yeah, I have a question: This whole thing you have going on with all these philosophers; do any of the boys ever provide an answer? What I mean is, do they ever get it right or do we just continue spinning our wheels for the next few years? What, exactly, is the point?"

He looked up from his notes and gave me a look like I had just insulted Mother Thayer. Then he left the podium and walked rather deliberately to my desk. No one, and I mean no one, looked up or uttered a word. My brother seminarians stared impassively at the floor as Fr. Thayer bellowed, "Dr. Bradley," he said (I should note that you knew you were in trouble when the professor referred to you by an academic title you didn't have), "the intrinsic point of the disciplined study of philosophy is *humility*. That *is* the goal. Just when you think you have mastered the secrets of the cosmos, I will alert you to the fact you have not even begun."

His delivery was straight out of John Houseman in the wonderful movie, *Paper Chase*. Properly chastised, I never again raised my hand in class to offer a smart ass question.

For every college seminarian, the final months at St. Joseph's are filled with tension as the application process to St. Patrick's — the major seminary — begins. Near the end of my final semester, the faculty offered their evaluation and recommendation for each candidate. They had three basic options:

1. Yes, the student is qualified to move on to St. Patrick's, which meant he possessed the academic skills necessary to complete seminary training.
2. No, the student is not qualified to move forward, which meant he was politely and respectfully shown the door to immediately begin the process of finding a "real job."
3. Yes, the student is qualified *with reservations*, which basically meant do not unpack your bags because you will be officially dismissed in short order...with kindness and love, of course.

That was it, those were the three possibilities. I had diligently kept my secret of occasional drinking and using to myself, so I was fairly confident I would be recommended for St. Patrick's. I had strictly followed the unofficial seminarian creed, which was to say nothing controversial and show up for everything on time and with a smile. Deep down, I had tremendous admiration for the priests and lay professors who taught us. They were totally dedicated and men and women of profound faith. I didn't want to disappoint them, but my overall focus was one of self-preservation; I liked living in the structure of the seminary and very much wanted to advance to St. Patrick's. Of course, I also wanted to keep drinking and using. As long as I could keep it in control, I knew I'd be fine.

The morning the letters arrived from St. Patrick's, and I noticed several classmates slumped in their rooms; their body language and teary eyes told me all I needed to know. As I walked to the mailroom, I wondered what I would do if I was rejected? I didn't think the airline would re-hire me, and I had no other job prospects lined up, so it was a rather long, slow walk to the mailroom.

When I picked up the letter, I walked outside into the bright sunshine. I figured if I wasn't deemed worthy to move on, I'd rather hear it in the warm outdoors than the cold marble hallways of St. Joseph's.

"Congratulations. You are accepted to St. Patrick's Seminary," was the first and only line of the letter I read. I was genuinely humbled because I knew there were well-qualified young men sitting in their rooms crying their eyes out, feeling rejected. I was also fully aware that *all of them* had lived more honorably and with more integrity than I had during our two years at St. Joseph's. I was flat out fortunate that the work I had put into my academic program had paid off. I also knew enough to keep a low but focused profile; always calm, but comfortable enough to be funny on cue. I knew exactly what the faculty wanted, and I delivered with calculated efficiency.

Looking back, I admit there probably should have been several serious reservations concerning my moving on to St. Patrick's. But since no one uttered a word or raised a question concerning my "readiness," I smiled politely and prepared to move on.

My old drinking buddy was not accepted to St. Patrick's. In fact, as the second year went by, he was resigned to dropping out regardless of the outcome. In the end, he chose not to apply and happily returned to his family.

14

St. Patrick's Seminary
and The Blessing of Fr. Robert Gavin

St Patrick's Seminary was a totally different ball game than St. Joseph's. The feeling among the faculty was that each seminarian had done his soul searching at St. Joseph's and was now prepared to begin the business of preparing for life as a priest. The assumption by everyone (including the seminarian) was that the discernment process was largely over, and it was now time to focus on the reality of serving as an ordained minister.

From the very beginning, I knew that the shenanigans I pulled at St. Joseph's would never happen at St. Patrick's. The students were older and more focused, and the whole atmosphere was seriously devoted to formation as a parish priest. Walking through the main door I could feel the difference. It was tangible. This was not a place to sneak out for a few beers during the week; it was time to see if serving as a priest was a real possibility for me.

The Rector of St. Patrick's was a wonderful man, Fr. Gerald "Jerry" Coleman. He was an experienced professor and administrator, and had lived and worked in a variety of parishes throughout the Archdiocese. Thus, he was comfortable in both the parish and academic worlds. In fact, he thrived in both. He was and is among the most respected priests in the Archdiocese of San Francisco.

The first order of business for the seminarian was to choose his Spiritual Director, which proved to be one of the most important decisions of my life. We were encouraged to spend the first week informally meeting and talking with each member of the faculty to get to know each other beyond the classroom.

From these brief discussions, we were allowed to choose the priest with whom we felt the most comfortable; the one we felt we could trust with our lives. It was one of the very few choices we made on our own, since the Spiritual Director has tremendous influence on the life of a seminarian. The relationship is sacred and confidential. The Spiritual Director does not even vote whether the seminarian is ready for ordination. I believe that, without qualification, it is the single most important relationship in the entire seminary system, since the relationship is built on trust and honesty. There is no gamesmanship or shading of the truth...for both seminarian and Director.

I hit a home run when I choose Fr. Robert (Bob) Gavin as my Spiritual Director. He was a beautiful man of faith with a gentle spirit that was filled with empathy and compassion. Lest anyone think they could pull a fast one and take advantage of his kindness or mistake his temperament for weakness...well, they were sadly mistaken. Fr. Bob could sense and obliterate nonsense in a New York minute, which happened to be where he was born and raised.

In his mid-sixties, Fr. Bob had a grey goatee and longish silver hair that flopped over his ears, and I wasn't sure if he was color blind, but he sure dressed like it. True to his nature, Fr. Bob had no regard for material possessions—none at all. He drove an older car, and couldn't care less about the latest in priest vestments. He was perfectly satisfied with his wide variety of clerical shirts, none which matched his pants and jackets. And the seminarians loved him. I used to call him my favorite Hippie priest.

In our initial meeting, we talked about the pitching staff for the Giants, the offensive needs of the 49ers, and the entire history of Notre Dame Football. Somewhere, somehow, I found myself, without even knowing it, completely opening up to him in ways I'd never done before. He had a realistic view of seminary life and priesthood—he didn't glamorize it or make it sound heroic; it was just one way of answering God's call and invitation to serve His people. I was impressed with his pragmatic, down to earth style, and I intuitively felt I could trust him.

What he did emphasize was the importance of developing a deep prayer life, saying, "Everything you say and do must begin through your interior prayer life; you have to constantly nurture it. That is the single most important thing you can do for yourself in the years you are here."

In addition, he took the pressure off grades by advising, "Study prayerfully; don't worry about your grades. The things you will learn here you will use in the parish and throughout your ministry. Try to internalize everything you learn, take it all in because you will use it to help someone when you get out there. You are not here to become a scholar, you are here to become a parish priest. Your prayer life will be the keys to your own happiness and peace and that, in turn, will make you a wonderful priest."

No truer words were ever spoken. Fr. Bob's focus was deeply rooted in the spiritual struggle for a sense of peace and understanding, and everything he said and did began with quiet prayer.

I noticed that Fr. Bob rarely used words like "success," or "accomplish." He preferred "serenity" or "service" when referring to our vocation and life mission. When all was said and done, they were the only things that really mattered—serenity in our relationship with God, and service to His people as an expression of our faith. What impressed me most about Fr. Bob is that he didn't just talk *about* ministry; he truly lived it in a humble, but joyful, way. I was moved by the way he never called attention to himself. Instead, he gently went about his ministry connecting with everyone he met.

I realized he was the person I'd been waiting to meet for a long time. If I were to make it to ordination and become a good and decent and honorable priest, Fr. Bob Gavin was the man I wanted with me as my Spiritual Director.

Perhaps it was a grace from God, but for some reason I poured out my entire life history the first time we formally sat down together. I held nothing back, and spoke from my heart. I shared the fun and the subsequent horror of my airline days, Steve's death, the lingering sadness and loss from losing Dad, my alcohol and drug abuse...everything. I think it was the first time I'd been completely honest with anyone regarding the mistakes in my life. I even shared my pattern of drinking while a student at St. Joseph's. Basically, I spilled my guts all over the room, and it felt really good to finally come clean. I had hidden from everyone, including myself, for such a long time, and I was tired of it.

I remember Fr. Bob—looking a tad pale—as I shared my brief history of life at St. Joseph's. At one point, he asked me, "What was the difference between your life at the airline the last year and your first year at St. Joseph's?"

My answer was frank. "Nothing. I slicked it up, but it was the same crazy stuff. Other than distance, I was leading the same basic life. It might have looked different on the surface, but it was the same game. I'm starting to wonder if it is simply part of who I am. It seems to be one of the things I'm quite good at. Even all the way back to the airline days, I should have been caught so many times, and I never was."

When I finished, he sat back, cleared his throat, and in a very gentle voice said, "Well, we all have something in our lives that pulls us away from God and ourselves. You are actually *lucky* because you can name what it is. Lots of people go through their entire lives without knowing what it is."

"Lucky?" Did he just say "lucky" in regards to my struggles? I had never considered myself *lucky* to have a problem with alcohol and using. Cursed maybe, but lucky? Hell no.

But unlike anyone I ever met in my life, Fr. Bob Gavin had a remarkable way of turning things around and asking me to slow down and take a good look from a different perspective. He actually said, "God brought you here, Joey (Bob is the only person in my entire life to ever call me Joey), so you can be a priest and teach others what you have learned. You will be a grace in our community, and when you're ordained, you will be a grace to those who suffer in your parish. You will understand situations that others won't. We need what you will bring."

Now, let's just pause and consider this for a moment: We were basically still in the "feeling out" process, still getting to know each other, and he was already referring to my addiction as a grace. In fact, he was referring to me as a grace from God. I shook my head wondering, *what is it with this guy, is* everything *a grace?* Turns out that in the spiritual world of Fr. Bob Gavin, just about everything *is* a grace because all things are centered and connected to God. Nothing happens on an island and everything is spiritually linked. I stared at him intently, and decided he was the most uniquely spiritual person I'd ever met. His world view spoke to me of Jesus, and I was in awe of him right from the beginning.

One thing was clear: Fr. Bob Gavin had a very different view of me than I had of myself. I remember wondering if he knew he was dealing with the best con artist in the building. I was the guy who was high as a kite during seminary midterm exams at St. Joseph's…and managed to keep it hidden from the entire community.

But Fr. Bob was adamant; he saw addiction, or anything similar, as a chance to grow *closer* to God. He felt that people in recovery had paid their dues and emerged with a unique perspective on God's love and mercy. He was so full of spiritual hope, and I wanted to catch and hold on to what he offered.

For my part, I admitted that I didn't feel I had control over my desires to drink and use, even though I wished I did. I also admitted that I believed God could help me and take those burdens away. I believed that Jesus understood my journey and was willing to intercede on my behalf. After all, I had always loved that Jesus had a soft spot for lost souls, and I humbly admitted to Fr. Bob that I was most assuredly one of them.

He gently but firmly encouraged me to make contact with a few seminarians who had similar stories to mine and would be willing to talk. I had never, ever, reached out to anyone for anything like this. In fact, the only people I reached out to were those who could keep the ride going.

"No one recovers on an island, Joey." Fr. Bob was convinced that surrounding myself with like-minded people, people who took their healing and recovery seriously, was going to be key to my future. In the past, even when first entering the college seminary, I seemed to always gravitate toward people who drank and used; now, I was going to reach out to an entirely different community.

When our first session ended, Fr. Bob asked if I wanted to pray with him. I remember looking over and saying, "Bob, I don't think I have ever admitted this to anyone, but I always knew down deep that alcohol, and all that accompanies it, will always have the potential to kick my ass. I can play it off for a while, but sooner or later I just know it will catch me, and I don't want to relive the loss of Steve or anyone else ever again. It's too damn painful, and I'm tired of it. It might sound cliché, but I am truly sick and tired of being sick and tired. "

And that was the day I realized that the game was up.

My classmates might have the luxury to enjoy a drink now and then, but I didn't. It just didn't work for me. I was tired of the lies and sneaking around trying to hide what I was doing. If I ever did make it as a priest, what was I going to do? Hide six packs of beer and interrupt parish meetings to run to my room for drink or toke of marijuana?

I wanted to reclaim a sense of integrity. I wanted to be a seminarian, not a fraud who had become quite the expert at covering up for himself. I wanted to be a genuine man who was real with his vows and promises. I wanted to end the charade. I wanted to become a priest who lived what he believed.

Fr. Bob and I prayed together that night in the privacy of his room, and the next morning I woke up and cleaned out my room. I still had a few beer cans and a tiny amount of marijuana tucked away. Surprisingly, it was quite emotional placing the beers in garbage cans and flushing the marijuana down the toilet. At St. Patrick's, the restrooms and showers were located at the end of each hallway, so they were available for anyone to use...I must have flushed the toilet twenty times to make sure all the evidence was gone.

15

Ego

Although it was certainly not the original intention, St. Patrick's became something of a rehab center for me, as well as a seminary. In retrospect, I probably should have temporarily withdrawn from the seminary and entered a rehab facility, but I believed I could work through it while remaining a student. I poured myself into the spiritual program at St. Patrick's, and I met with Fr. Bob almost every week. I began pursuing sobriety on a serious basis for the first time since I began using after Dad's death. After his passing, I quickly developed an uncontrollable urge to put anything into my system that would numb my feelings and emotions. I would go to any length to avoid facing reality. Rather, I would place myself and others at risk rather than be completely honest with myself. Instead of confronting what was going on in my life, I would flee to the sanctuary of alcohol or anything I could get my hands on.

I wanted to know why I had this tendency to run away when things didn't go my way and seek comfort in a chemical. With Fr. Bob leading weekly discussions, I dug beneath the surface and quickly accepted one of the main reasons I drank and used was to fit in and become part of a community that shared life together. Using drugs opened the doors to a lot of friendships in my life. It was fun to fit in with a group I'd always watched from a distance. It felt good to be part of them as they were part of me. I liked the emotional connection almost as much as the high itself.

But while a desire to fit in was definitely a factor, I knew there was a deeper one, and it was harder to admit. The culprit was my over the top, completely out of control EGO. When I was happy...when I was sad...when I was hurt...when I failed...when I succeeded...I would drink or use. What was the operative word? "I" or "Me" or "Mine"...pick one, but it was all directed to the same theme of "Self."

Very slowly, and relying on Fr. Bob to steer the course of the discussion, I came to the grim realization that *I* was the one behind my own struggles. It wasn't God, or church, or anyone else...I brought it on myself. For years, I blamed everyone and everything, so it was quite a revelation to humbly admit I fell by my own hand.

I'd always had this pattern that when something didn't go my way exactly how and when I wanted, I would fight like hell to force it to happen. And when it still wouldn't go the way I wanted, I would get angry and bitter, and wrap myself up in my "poor me" feelings and hide in a bottle. As time evolved, I would hide in the bottle for longer and longer periods of time until the bottle became the essence of my life.

My own ego was killing me. I felt embarrassed admitting it, but I also felt strangely liberated. It was good to finally speak the truth without trying to cover up and hide from it. I'd spent so many years hiding from the obvious that it was a genuine relief to acknowledge I had no defense against the need to drink and use. It felt good to let it come out.

Gradually, the focus of my prayer started to shift. Instead of offering the Lord a laundry list of things I wanted, I actually asked for the strength to know and accept His will in my life. For me, that was one hellacious spiritual change.

Each morning when I woke up in my room at St. Patrick's, I would begin by offering the Serenity Prayer:

God grant me the serenity to accept the things I cannot change,
The courage to change the things I can,
And the wisdom to know the difference.

It was a whole lot different than greeting each day at the airlines or college seminary with a cold one, ready to fight for my way or no way. Slowly, it began to make a difference in my prayer, my vocation, and my life. Thus began the process of surrendering my will to God, and I began to accept that each time I fought to uphold my will, it led to unmitigated disaster. This truly was a process because, at least for me, such a radical change in priorities and perspectives didn't happen overnight; it took time and patience—two virtues I was not blessed with during my drinking and using career.

16

Surrender

I was raised in a family who loved sports. I was taught to play with aggression—clean, but aggressive. It's how all the neighborhood kids played. The one cardinal sin you never broke (at least in our home) was to quit, or give up...or, dare I say it...*surrender*. Anything but that, and I mean *anything*. Surrender was the ultimate sign of weakness. In the world of neighborhood sports, you were mocked for giving up.

So when I first heard the word used in relation to recovery from addiction, I literally stopped in my tracks. Did it mean quit? Did it mean run away? Did it mean I was too soft and weak to handle the problem? Just what did it mean? I soon learned from Fr. Bob and my new buddies in recovery that it was the difference between living and dying, and the single most courageous act I could offer if I wanted to stop the madness in my life and move forward.

Until then, I had never, ever heard "surrender" and "courage" in the same sentence. But it seemed that the most significant step was to literally surrender my life into God's hands and let God do for me what I couldn't do for myself. I had to let go of my own ego's tired attempt to control what I could not control. It made frightening sense.

I remember telling Fr. Bob that I'd once heard the saying that insanity was doing the same thing over and over again, each time expecting a different result. "If that's true, I am definitely insane when it comes to drinking and using because I've been doing the same thing for years."

My new pals told me over long lunches and coffee meetings that, in their humble opinion, my best hope for survival was to literally turn the whole damn mess over to God and promise to only live out of His spiritual wisdom. I could fight my drinking forever and nothing would work until I reached the point of surrender. They even used Fr. Bob's favorite word to describe the moment of giving it over: It would be a *Grace.*

I considered it very seriously; I mean, no one wants to admit we are beaten. I wanted to stay in the fight and pull myself out of the hole, but maybe, just maybe, all these people weren't wrong. Maybe they were right, and I was wrong. Maybe it really was time to follow their experienced advice.

So, I did. I actually did it.

I was finally ready and offered complete surrender to God on His terms. I hit both knees and literally begged God to accept my surrender. *"Please take this intense yearning to drink and use away from me. Please. I just can't stop it. I try. I try and I try, and I just cannot pull it off. I am an accomplished liar and bullshitter, but I cannot talk my way out of it. I am defeated, and I ask you to please save me and take this crazy need away from me. Please."*

I waved the white flag of surrender alone in my room at St. Patrick's Seminary. And when I finished my plea, I felt it was a moment of grace, an epiphany. My surrender was, in fact, a victory.

I started to get better. I started to really get clean. I started to get sober.

17

Meetings: New Perspectives

One afternoon, I knocked on the door of an older seminarian who had been very public about his past struggles and had a good reputation for helping others. I looked into his clear eyes and almost whispered, "Um, I, uh, hear you attend meetings?"

He smiled. "Yes, several days a week. Are you a friend of Bill W.?"

I nodded. "If you don't mind, I would like to join you some day."

"How about today? There's an afternoon meeting not far from here, so we can chat on the way over."

That afternoon he handed me what is commonly known as the "Big Book" of Alcohol Anonymous. "Read it, pray about it. You might find your own story in the ones shared in this book. Follow the steps, and come to meetings. Let God do the work with you and for you."

I didn't know it that day, but he was to become my sponsor in A.A. and walk with me through *the* major change in my life.

My first surprise about life in A.A. meetings was that there were several other seminarians present and comfortably waiting for the start of the meeting. They knew lots of people in attendance, so I figured they had to be veterans. I felt very much at home listening to a speaker talk about his story, which didn't seem that much different from mine. Our struggles were eerily similar, and I could relate to his emotion.

After the meeting, my soon-to-be sponsor invited to me to join the other seminarians for coffee at the local Starbucks. I enjoyed everything about it—the prayerful spirit, the brutal honesty, and the beautiful sense of camaraderie. When we returned to St. Patrick's, I was on a natural high and filled with gratitude. I could look myself in the mirror again.

Sensing that I might leap forward too quickly, my new pal called that night and warned to me to take it slow, literally one day at time; sometimes, one minute or second at a time. "We alcoholics tend to jump into things, Joe, so go real slow and be gentle and patient with yourself. I'll see you at tomorrow's meeting…oh, and keep reading the book, it has the answers we are all looking for."

Be patient and move slowly— wow, I had never been either with anyone. I was always full throttle with no hesitation or thought for any of the risks. But I found that the meetings had an effect on my prayer and my life. I began to slow down the pace and take a longer and deeper look around me. I saw, for maybe the first time, just how remarkably fortunate I was. My family had never given up on me, and I was now surrounded by clean and sober people willing to help and support. And despite all odds, I was living comfortably and happily in a Catholic seminary. I was much more fortunate than I deserved.

One day, while walking the seminary grounds, a fellow seminarian who had several years of sobriety said, "Joe, there are only two things you must acknowledge and believe to have real peace in your life: 1) Yes, there is an all knowing, all powerful God. 2) You ain't it."

That was it

That was the key to recovery, happiness, and internal peace. I needed to let God be God. That meant I had to stop trying to manipulate His will and spirit. I needed to continue developing my prayer to feel His presence within me, and simply follow His call—without challenging it. By living this way, I would be granted a 24-hour reprieve from how I lived before. I felt it was more than worth it.

Eventually, a well-respected priest joined us at our meeting. At first I was shocked to see him, but it symbolically drove home the point that the disease can and does affect anyone. Really good people with high integrity can fall into its trap. His presence humbled me, and taught me yet another lesson—no one is immune, and we can all become its prey.

18

Honest Admissions

After being clean and sober for several months, I thought it was long past time to come clean with my Vocation Director. He deserved the truth. I called him at the Chancery Office and set an appointment the next time he was scheduled to visit St. Patrick's. Despite being nervous during the application process for the college seminary, I was honest with him in our interviews. However, after few months, I wondered if I'd underestimated the depth of the problem.

At the time, I'd left him feeling that my addictions were under control, and while I might have thought so, they clearly were not. They were actually getting worse each day. Regardless of the potential consequences, I needed to be honest with him about changes I was making. My sobriety depended on rigorous honesty, and that meant no longer taking the easy way out. It was something of a bottom for me. I was out of charm, out of lies, and out of excuses. It was time to face up to what I had become.

The lessons I learned through the loss of Steve had definitely rocked my world, but with time, I'd felt I could get past them and control what I was doing. It just wasn't true. I had no control whatsoever. I was tired. It was time to face facts and speak the truth.

When Fr. Bruce Dreier arrived at the seminary, I met him outside the chapel where I had prayed to accept God's will in regards to our conversation. I spoke honestly and admitted to drinking and using while a seminarian at St. Joseph's Seminary and concluded by admitting my own shame and discussing my commitment to A.A. and recovery. With permission, I even offered the name of my sponsor.

I was nervous that Fr. Bruce would (rightfully) inform the Archbishop, who had the power to have me removed from St. Patrick's, and I was also worried that such information would somehow get out into the seminary community and become fuel for the legendary seminary gossip machine. But I wrote off the fears as testimony to my own ego and sensitivities getting in the way of doing the right thing.

In the end, Fr. Bruce was a rock, and supported me when he didn't have to. I still remember him saying, "Joe, this isn't a place to hide, and I'm glad to hear you're working on what you need to—it will make you a better priest. You continue attending your meetings and let's keep in touch with how things are progressing. You have my prayers and complete support."

I spent five years at St. Patrick's and Fr. Bruce Dreier never wavered in his support. Neither did the seminarians I attended meetings with, and others who eventually learned the truth of my struggles with drugs and alcohol. After years of lying and deception—even as a seminarian—I did not deserve their support, but by the grace of God they still offered it.

I would have never made it without them. Left to my own ways, I would have slipped back into past ways of life. Something would have come along to challenge or tweak my emotions, and I would have been right back where I first started. I suppose different people can attain sobriety in different ways, but for me it was faith in God and faith in His people. I am forever grateful to those who helped me, when I was quite unable to help myself.

19

Ministry while at St. Patrick's

The process of becoming sober not only affected my prayer life, it also affected my sense of ministry. I didn't look at the world through a clerical collar, but through the eyes of a former drunk and user. The only ambition I had was to remain sober...at any price.

I brought that genuine sense of humility to every pastoral situation I experienced. My goal was to help and serve, to walk the journey with parishioners, not to tell anyone what to do or how to think. Frankly, I didn't give a damn about how many degrees I worked to attain, or what my academic reputation was...none of that mattered. I was a former drunk who was only one drink, one slip, from falling back into the abyss of darkness and loss. I only wanted to be there for someone else with similar struggles. Nothing more and nothing less.

At St. Patrick's, each seminarian was assigned to a parish or institution each weekend. My second year, I was assigned to work in an adult education program at a wonderfully active parish in San Francisco, along with the opportunity to work on the Chaplain's staff at San Quentin Prison.

It was only a part time job, basically filling in when extra help was needed, but it was a powerful experience. Each Sunday, Mass was held in a concrete building that was large enough to hold about seventy-five inmates. To a person, the inmates were respectful the minute they entered the church. It was like they left their troubles on the yard or the tiers, and entered the only sacred place in the entire institution.

My role was to occasionally help with communion, along with chatting with the inmates at the conclusion of the Mass. There was something of a picnic area immediately in front of the chapel and we'd sit and visit for a brief time before the inmates were called to lunch.

One afternoon, an inmate called me over and said, "Joe, ya just gotta tell me, why do you want to be a priest? I don't get it…and no disrespect, but I don't see it."

I couldn't help but smile. "You aren't the only one."

The inmate offered a hearty laugh. "Honest, man, I just don't see it."

"I don't want to bore you because it's a long story."

"Hell, Joe, take your time … I've got another ten years."

I decided to spare none of the morbid and embarrassing details, and gave him a full and honest account of my spiritual journey, complete with all the regrets. As I spoke, he would nod his head and even smile from time to time…we were on the same page.

When I finished, he looked at me for a long time, and then, with utmost seriousness, he said, "I get it. I really do. And I wish you all the luck in the world. But do me a favor, when you get out there…away from all the schooling…keep it real, right? I mean, your story, you gotta keep it real. Don't smooth it over after you become a priest. Instead, talk it just like you did today with me."

In the following months, we sat together each time I came for Mass at San Quentin; just two thirty-something guys talking sports and church. He was dressed in blue denim jeans and jacket, and I in my black, clerical shirt—but we both had way more in common than anyone might have thought. Wherever you are today my friend, I hope you are OK, and I hope you're pleased that I never stop trying to "keep it real."

I remember coming back to St. Pat's after one of my infrequent visits to the prison and telling Fr. Bob and my new "recovery" pals about some of the men I met during the visit. None of us failed to realize that we had a lot in common with our incarcerated brothers; alcohol and drug use had also been the source of our problems as well. I remember Mom once saying, "There but for the grace of God go I."

Indeed.

When I think of nights I drove home under the influence, buying drugs on airport property, and stealing everything in sight, I know damn well that could have been me sitting on the other side of that prison bench. I will always know that. I will never forget how close I came.

For the rest of my years at St. Patrick's, I would end the night with a prayer of thanksgiving for my sobriety, and I'd offer a special one for those still in the darkness. I would also pray for the inmates in prison, that, through the grace of God, they would find their way into recovery and taste the light of freedom from addiction.

20

Ordination as a Transitional Deacon

In 1990, after seven years in the seminary, I, along with my classmates, applied to be ordained "Transitional Deacons." This basically means that we have earned the recommendation from the faculty at St. Patrick's and that we promise to see our vocation through to ordination as a priest. This is a major event because the rite includes a public promise to our Bishop that we will follow God's call to become a priest, and to live a chaste/celibate life. Bottom line: We promise not turn to back.

The Bishop is the spiritual leader of the diocese, and is responsible for the placement and guidance of his priests. Since I believe he is an instrument of God's will, I had no problem humbling myself to pledge obedience to him.

Obedience: Hmm, not exactly the strong point of my life. Got me in a whole lot of trouble as a younger man. But now, with some quality sobriety behind me, I was prepared to offer it to my Bishop with a pure and clear heart. It was part of following God's will.

Celibacy: The accepted belief at St. Patrick's was that, by the time you arrived, you had *already* been living a celibate life for several years, and of course, that commitment would remain throughout your seminary career…no exceptions.

The truth is, for me, I had never really experienced a physically intimate relationship before entering seminary. That's not to say that I was never in love or gave my heart away, but I was never in a serious, committed relationship. I was certainly never close to entering into sacramental marriage.

Sexual intimacy was usually a matter of flat out luck. More often than not, it was the aftermath of a party or social gathering among acquaintances. It was usually beer and drug-fueled and, by mutual agreement, forgotten the following morning.

For some reason the relationships just never seemed to work. Like most people consumed with using, I had a gift for sabotaging relationships that had the potential for love. When reduced to being the proverbial friend, I would passively accept my fate once I had a variety of substances in me. Although I had close women friends, I always knew I was destined to head off in a very different direction. Inexplicably, it was a feeling that rang true to the core of my being.

Even during the wildest days of rage (and regret), I wondered if, somehow, I would reconcile with the Lord and find my way back. I would deny it to family and friends, but I think the call was still there. Ultimately, I believe it was my fate and destiny.

Had providence been different, I probably would have been one of those soccer dads whose life revolves around his family, buying into the whole package of BBQ's, baseball games, and family vacations. But while such a life had its attraction, I knew my eventual the path led to seminary and priesthood, though I never anticipated causing quite as much hell on the way.

As each summer passed during my seven-year stay in the seminary, more and more of my classmates dropped out; most of their own accord, some by way of faculty recommendation. Had I not been sober, I have no idea what I would have done. Chances are that I would have left for one reason or another. While considering the celibate commitment, there was one fact that often preempted all other thoughts: As a young man, I had never been in a relationship that didn't involve drinking and/or using, so there were times in seminary when I wondered what it might be like to find a life partner while sober. I remember talking to Fr. Bob about it and sharing the concern with my classmates during days of retreat and reflection.

Fr. Bob was typically gentle but firm, and bluntly suggested that if I thought I was missing something in my life, I needed to take a leave and go out and experience it. "Joey, don't get ordained still wondering if it's for you. You'll only get disillusioned and bitter that something or someone might still be out there for you. Take whatever you're thinking deep into your prayer and see where God is calling you."

I had long since learned to follow Fr. Bob's insights and suggestions, so I made it a priority in my prayer. It slowly occurred to me that my real fear was loneliness. I didn't want to become some old, bitter priest whose loneliness got the best of him. I thought that was more frightening than living as a celibate.

I didn't hesitate to share my fears with Fr. Bob on one of our long walks around the seminary grounds. I told him that although there were lots of times I was alone in the seminary, I had never really felt lonely because there was always someone to call or visit. But I wondered how it might be in a parish where I might not know anyone. Loneliness could be a real problem for me because I feared falling back to old ways just to avoid the feeling.

He reminded me that it would be important to cultivate appropriate friendships and to join a priest support group through the Archdiocese. Fr. Bob put great emphasis on the importance of forming a supportive community. "Don't be the Lone Ranger. Don't try and go it alone because that's how guys, even really good guys, get in trouble."

Fr. Bob offered a few general examples of those who lost their way because their world became "too small," and they literally let their room collapse all around them. He added, "You'll need a good, healthy, social life, or things will close in on you. The result is that you'll seek comfort in unhealthy ways."

As our walk came to a close, I paused. "I have one more question, what happens if I meet someone in a parish setting and, without intentionally seeking it, fall in love with the person? I mean, does that ever happen?"

Fr. Bob smiled and patted my shoulder, "Joey, you will be working with good people all the time in a very public setting and the truth is, it is bound to happen at some point during your life as a priest."

I smiled back, "Damn, Bob, that would be just my luck to find sober love as a priest."

In the end, I felt that God had brought me to the seminary, and I was ready to publically voice my promise to live in obedience to my Bishop, and as a celibate man for the rest of my life. I felt at peace with it and ready to be ordained a Transitional Deacon.

I loved my life as a Deacon. It was my first real opportunity to offer the sacraments and preach at Sunday Mass. As a Deacon, I entered into people's lives during their most happy and joyful moments, and also at their saddest. One day I would celebrate the baptism of a baby, and the next help with the funeral of a loved one. For me, the ministry was pure grace.

Several months after being ordained a Deacon, I received a phone call from my Vocation Director, Fr. Bruce Dreier. He had been with me through some dark days, but now was calling with good news: Archbishop John R. Quinn, was prepared to ordain me a Catholic Priest, April 13th, 1991.

Unbelievable.

Thanks be to our God of mercy and forgiveness.

21

Ordination as a Catholic Priest

In the months leading up to my ordination, I was allowed to choose a specific scriptural verse that best defined my journey to priesthood. The verse or passage would be quoted on my ordination prayer card and formal invitation cards. I prayed about it and came up with the verse that best described my spiritual journey:

"My grace is enough for you,
For power is made perfect in weakness.
Therefore, I will proudly boast of my weakness,
That Christ may dwell in me,
For it is when I am weak, that I am strong."
(2 Cor:12:9-12)

The passage was from St. Paul's letter to the church in Corinth, and I believe he was referring to his ministry. I loved his comment, "…For it is when I am weak that I am strong."

It summed up my entire life. Had I never finally attained the grace to surrender my life into His hands, there is no doubt I would still be floundering about drinking and using, and lying and cheating. I never would have found happiness or a sense of peace. I looked at my entire ordination as a celebration of God's healing, mercy, and forgiveness. I don't mean to sound overdramatic or give a false sense of humility, but I felt remarkably unworthy of the calling to serve as a priest. Yet, I felt incredible joy and happiness, like I was coming home from a long, laborious hike through a scary mountain range, only to finally look up and see the path leading home.

The morning of my ordination, I met my younger brother John at a basketball court near Mom's house and played some hoops while we paused to laugh about the rather violent scrimmages we'd played against each other as kids. When it was time to get ready, I left early and drove to Holy Cross Cemetery where Dad and several of my relatives rest peacefully. I remember bowing on the wet grass at Dad's grave and thanking him for his spiritual presence throughout my life, especially in the dark days. I felt that Dad supported my vocation from heaven, and I wanted a few moments alone with him before driving to St. Mary's Cathedral of the Assumption.

When I arrived at St. Mary's, I walked around the magnificent cathedral and chatted with friends I hadn't seen in a long, long time. I thanked an old airline pal, who noted, "There was no way I was going to miss this. Now I can say I've actually witnessed a miracle."

I believe he was right.

There was one part of the Mass that will stay with me forever. It was a ritual within the Ordination Rite called, "The Litany of Saints." I was invited to lie prostrate on the floor while the Cathedral Choir and the entire assembly prayerfully sang the names of the saints and asked for their spiritual guidance and intercession for my priesthood. Their beautiful voices filled the Cathedral with faith and hope. I remember it as if it were yesterday. I saw everyone.

With my eyes closed but heart open, I saw everyone who helped lead me to this moment. I saw Dad so clearly I felt I could touch him. He wore that knowing smile he often shared when he knew we were up to something. He looked so peaceful and content, that I was moved to tears. They rained down across my face and over my arms and landed on the marble floor near the altar.

I saw Mom behind me, and she looked equally at peace. I couldn't help but remember her words of faith that terrible night of Steve's accident. She never gave up on me, and now I was being ordained a priest in the faith she taught me.

I also saw my sister and brother, Maureen and John, with their families. They, too, never gave up on me and always reflected the models of faith and encouragement. Whatever path I was on, they never wavered with love and support. I know I had to have frustrated them many times, but they never turned their backs on me.

And of course, I saw my old friend Steve. He looked at me on my belly on the Cathedral floor and said, "Dude, even God is surprised."

I think I even saw the shadow of Agent Dave, the corporate security officer sent to investigate me at the airport. He looked rather stunned, and who could blame him? He saw me at my absolute worst. Agent Dave, wherever you are, God bless you. Thank you for your attempt to wake me up from the choices I was making.

I saw aunts and uncles who had long since passed, but had convened to see me on this happiest day of my life. And I saw an old friend, David Fontenot, a young man I sponsored for Confirmation, who died tragically from cancer.

I was deeply honored at those who came—both living and gone—to help celebrate a life that was lost and had been found.

In the weeks before the ordination, I was allowed to choose a priest to help vest me so, of course, I asked Fr. Bob, who graciously accepted. As he prepared to place the sacred vestments over my head, he winked and flashed his most mischievous smile and whispered, "OK, dear Joey, I know you are ready."

I couldn't respond, as tears again flooded my face and I mumbled an incoherent, "Thank you, Bob, I am so grateful to you."

I gave communion to Mom and all my family, after which friends and relatives came up to receive the sacrament. The hope and dream I had as a young man of becoming a priest came true, and God made me a priest almost in spite of myself.

22

First Mass

The following day, I offered my first Mass at St. Mark's Parish, where I thanked my family for their love and support, and the faculty and staff at St. Patrick's Seminary. Whether I had been ordained a priest or not, St. Patrick's saved my life because they molded my spirit, body, and emotions into a functioning minister of the Gospel, and they did it with passion, love, and faith.

St Mark's brought me face to face with my addictions to the point where I ran out of places to hide. The process of Spiritual Direction with an experienced Director was the lifesaver for me. I owe my life and priesthood to Fr. Bob because he got through to me when no one else could. He gave me an image of faith—real faith—that has stayed with me to this day. He modeled what priesthood is all about, and he did it more by what he did than what he said. He lived the Gospel every day of his life, and his influence will live on in my life forever. Twenty-one years after my ordination, there isn't a day that goes by that I don't think of Fr. Bob and the lessons he taught me.

Ironically, the Gospel for my first Mass was the story of Doubting Thomas. In fact, I couldn't have planned it any better because there wasn't anyone who related to Thomas as a young man more than I.

I began my sermon by saying, "As many of you know all too well, I wasn't always close to God, but I believe God was always close to me, even when I didn't want God in my life. This first Mass of my priesthood is a celebration of God's healing and love and forgiveness."

At a certain point, we took a moment of silence to pray for those still out in the darkness of anger, resentment and addictions.

In the end, it was a wonderful celebration. Before the final blessing, I took a quiet moment to let it all sink in by looking around the church and thanking God for rescuing me from myself, and allowing me to serve as a Catholic priest.

Postscript: Several years after I was ordained a priest, Fr. Bob Gavin died of heart failure. He'd retired from St. Patrick's and moved to a retirement home in Maryland, where he died several months later. Fr. Bob's entire life was devoted to helping people like me graduate from the seminary and function as a diocesan priest. I believe that when his work was complete, God simply called him home. Rest in Peace, Fr. Bob. I love you, and I will never forget all you did for me.

The Third Gift:
A New Heart

23

St. Charles Parish

One of my first assignments as a priest was at St. Charles Parish in San Carlos, about forty miles south of San Francisco. It was a large, upper middle class parish that was shepherded by Fr. John Ryan, a wonderful pastor with an Irish brogue that exposed his birth in Tipperary, Ireland. St. Charles was his first assignment as a pastor, and he led the parish with patience, faith, and understanding. He loved a good game of golf and became quite knowledgeable about American sports. We hit it off immediately.

Within the first three months of service as Associate Pastor, I came down with a terrible cold that quickly developed into pneumonia. It was severe enough to require several days of hospitalization. When the hospital doctors noted our family history of heart disease, they ran a battery of tests and were pleased to announce that my heart was in "fine shape," although my blood pressure was quite high - 140/100, which was high enough to begin medication to bring it down to a more acceptable level. I really never gave it much thought before, but this news enticed me to make a determined effort to embrace a healthier diet and begin more serious exercise.

Throughout the year, I kept getting colds and flu, and spent significant time in and out of my primary care physician's office. She concluded that, in addition to high blood pressure, I had developed symptoms of adult asthma. I was prescribed a host of inhalers and was eventually prescribed prednisone, a steroid, to reduce the swelling in my airways.

There was too much to do in my new job, so I didn't waste much time thinking about my health. I wanted to make a good impression on the people of the parish, and passed off my constant colds and flu as the result of over extending my work.

Mom felt quite differently, and she was always calling me out on my never-ending cough. Constantly clearing my throat was a nuisance, but I didn't feel it was anything to worry about. I just needed to slow down my pace, and things would be fine...only if that damn cough would ease up.

Illness aside, I loved serving as a priest. I absolutely loved every minute of it. I loved offering Mass, visiting the sick and their families, and participating in all the functions that make for an active parish. As a new priest, I enjoyed wonderful support from the community, and I was deeply touched at how they went out of their way to make me feel welcome.

At night in my room, I would thank God for such a blessing. From a pot smoking, beer drinking, coke head, to a Catholic priest. Damn, that really *is* a miracle.

Sunday mornings I packed the house. People knew what they were getting when it was my turn to preach. I was going all out. No holding back or backing down. I entered every Mass with the full intention of blowing the doors off the hinges with my enthusiasm and joy. There were times I would actually pinch myself that this was really happening. I was really a priest, preaching at Sunday Mass in front of two hundred and fifty people.

I would work myself into a lather of sweat while delivering my homily and, I don't know about anyone else in the church, but I had a blast. I never studied films of traditional, influential preachers. No way. Instead, I poured over old VCR tapes of Robin Williams because I was captivated at his ability to charm his audience while rocking the house with his wit and lightning-fast delivery. I never used notes or preached from the pulpit. Instead, I would grab a microphone off the stand and charge down the middle aisle into the center of the church and let loose.

I always prepared my homilies with a Bible and the newspaper, searching for anything that might be socially relevant to our community. I was determined that, even if I blew the homily to pieces, people knew I was into the message. I think people enjoyed my efforts. I mean, let's face it, my beloved Catholic Church could sure use homilies that don't invite peaceful slumber.

I kept my sobriety as my most treasured grace because I felt everything revolved around it. The blessing of my priesthood and the joy of serving in an active, supportive community kept me humble because I knew all too well that I would always be capable of falling. Only God's remarkable grace and sharing my past with people who had the same struggle could keep me on the straight and narrow. I prayed every morning and evening, maintained contacts in A.A., and attended meetings on a regular basis.

I found a great sponsor who had no association with the church. I thought it an important step because I wanted someone who could objectively call me out if I was heading for trouble. I appreciated how tough it could be for a sponsor to challenge his priest, so I sought out someone with whom I could be brutally honest and who could respond in the same manner.

During my second year as a priest, I received a grim reminder of the cost of falling back into my old ways after a priest friend called to tell me that one of our brothers was using again. Even though he had left the seminary, he was still a friend.

I picked up my friend and we drove directly to the address he had been given. We found our old buddy in the apartment he shared with a roommate. I was hit with the smell; like my old room at St.Joseph's. It was terrible. It was even worse to see him in such a state because he had been so good to me when I first got sober. We'd gone to meetings together and shared our thoughts over coffee. I'd foolishly assumed that since he was in the program, he would be fine. Instead, I was stunned at his condition. On a much deeper sense, I saw the stark reality of what drinking and using will ultimately lead to...for people like my old buddy and me.

I had never seen anyone fall away and slip back into drinking and using and, frankly, he scared me. We helped clean him up and made a few calls before making our way home. On the ride back to St. Charles, we both looked at each other, knowing full well that one bad move, one slip backwards, and that poor guy could be us.

It's a lesson I still think of on a daily basis.

24

Charlie's Angels — Youth Group Ministry

After I'd had some time to find my way around the parish, Fr. Ryan asked if I would take over the Confirmation Program and become the parish director of Youth Ministry. The sacrament of Confirmation was offered to high school students in their sophomore year. Getting fifteen and sixteen year-old kids, whose schedules were already overloaded, to come out to church on a Wednesday night was not always an easy task. They had to have a good reason to attend the classes or they would simply not come.

The spiritual roots of the Sacrament of Confirmation can be traced back to Pentecost—when Jesus appeared to His disciples after His resurrection and assured them of His spiritual presence as they moved forward to spread the good news of healing and faith. Jesus promised to be with them until the end of time. I always thought it was a beautiful vision of trust—not the disciple's trust in Jesus, but Jesus' trust in them. After all, these were the same fellas who bailed on Him at the first sign of trouble. I always thought it was much more a measure of Jesus' profound trust in His people, than our trust in Him. The Sacrament of Confirmation is a celebration of that same trust; we believe that Jesus' spirit continues to lead, guide, and inspire us to share in the mission of building His kingdom.

Now all that is well and fine, but as most parents and *all* priests know, very few—check that—*practically none of the kids wanted to be there*. In fact, with very few exceptions, they were only there under the false assumption that they had to be confirmed to (later) be married in the church.

Thus, my single biggest challenge of teaching Confirmation to a group of high school teenagers was "inspiration." I wanted to give them a reason to believe, a reason to see that there was something at stake in holding on to our faith.

One night, without really planning to do so, I opened up and shared my story with the kids. I think it's safe to say that the kids had *never* heard a priest use words or phrases like, cocaine, marijuana, stealing, police, corporate investigation, a car accident that resulted in the death of a friend, and refusal to pray or enter a church, as part of a vocation pitch. When I finished speaking, you could hear a pin drop. Then, all of a sudden, every hand in the room went up because the kids had loads of questions. As I looked out at their youthful faces, I remembered the words of my mentor, Fr. Bob Gavin, "Joey, this is why God brought you to us ..."

That class was one of our very few that didn't end exactly on time. We actually went way over our time limit. One of the kids asked, "What saved you?" I responded that it was a group of people who helped, and a loving, healing, and forgiving God. I made it clear that it took both to bring me out of the darkness and into the light.

From that night forward, everything about our class changed; the teenage students opened up and anything they wanted to discuss was open for dialogue. I think they liked the format because we actually added students to our roster; some even came from different parishes to participate in our discussions. On a personal level, it taught me that youngsters will respond and participate if they sense a connection that's real. If they feel free to share their thoughts and concerns without penalty, they will show up in droves.

I decided we needed to up the ante and form a youth group that might do some work in the community...maybe even outside it. Through the local Presbyterian Church, I learned about a wonderful faith-based, nondenominational group called "Amor Ministry," who ran a program in Mexico. They invited high school students to come down for a week and help build homes for people who were living on the streets.

I met with Fr. Ryan and asked his permission to organize such a trip. At first he was nervous, but he didn't say no, so I made my pitch. I said, "John, we will accomplish more in one week in Mexico working with the poor than five hundred classes on Confirmation. Our kids have no idea what's out there in the world. They think everyone lives like we do in San Carlos. This experience will stun them into realizing there is more than the comfortable parish we live in.

"We can talk all day to them...hell, we do...and we don't really accomplish much. But a week in the middle of nowhere with only our faith and each other will create memories that will stay with them a lifetime. I promise I can do this. These kids are only here at Confirmation because Mommy and Daddy make them, so it's up to us to change the conditions. A trip like this will change their lives and open new doors for their faith to grow."

To his everlasting credit, Fr. John Ryan approved the trip. There are damn few pastors who would trust a priest with one year of service to organize such a trip. Most would deny the request as too dangerous, and then spend the next year whining about why their teenage students were not involved in their parish community.

With Fr. John's approval, we made plans to bring a group of suburban kids from sheltered backgrounds to a poor village in Mexico for a week of service. We would live among the people, sleep in tents, prepare our own food, and take bucket showers of cold water. In short, we would experience life as we simply could not imagine.

Amor Ministry would provide the raw materials to build a small home—four walls with a tiny window, and a roof—for a family who had previously been living on the streets. In order to have that secure feeling of pride and ownership, the family would help us build their new home. We were there to serve and help in the process.

I would need a fairly large number of adult chaperones and at least one person with elementary skills in how to build a home. Initially, I planned to bring no more than fifteen or so teenagers for the mission. In the end, we wound up bringing about twenty-five people for our first "Mission to Mexico Trip."

In the weeks leading up to the trip, I developed another cold and, once again, it slipped into pneumonia. I was concerned enough that my primary care doctor sent me to a cardiologist. He cleared me to go on the trip, but noted that I had something of an irregular heartbeat, which meant that my heart would not maintain a steady beat. It would either beat too fast or too slow; once in a while it would actually skip a beat as well. Since the trip was fast approaching and we would be living in the middle of nowhere for a week, the cardiologist scheduled an angioplasty procedure to ensure that my arteries were clear.

With a family history just loaded with premature death due to heart disease, I was more than a little concerned. However, the results of the angioplasty procedure were pretty good, so I was allowed to go with the promise of checking back when we arrived home.

True to form, I failed to make the follow up appointment. Subconsciously, I didn't want to know if something was really wrong. Once again, in the face of potential turmoil, I chose not to look.

Where I was afraid to look at my own life, I was more than eager that everything be right for our Mexico trip. I suggested to our youth group that we should choose a name for ourselves, preferably something connected to the name of our parish. One night I left our meeting to preside at a funeral vigil and told the kids to have a name ready when I returned. After two hours of intense dialogue and prayerful reflection, "Charlie's Angels" was born.

25

Service in Mexico with Charlie's Angels

The day before we left, I attended a wonderful recovery meeting, and came home to offer Mass for the youngsters, their families, and our chaperones. I prayed for patience and understanding with our young and excited kids, and for the courage to accept God's way and will throughout our little adventure.

We received tremendous support from our parish community. Parents and couples without children made generous donations to our financial needs. It was apparent people understood that the best way to inspire youngsters in the ways of faith was to offer them a way to participate. During homilies, I would preach that this was not a social visit, but was a journey of faith, and we were there to fulfill Jesus' call to serve those less fortunate than ourselves. It was going to be hard work, but the payoff would be offering a home to people who, at this very moment, did not have one.

The good people of Amor Ministry made it clear to me that the real goal of the mission trip was for a young and impressionable group of teenagers to encounter Jesus in the poverty of a nameless village just a days' drive from where we live.

The day we left for Mexico, Fr. Ryan blessed the vans and offered a prayer for our safety. Privately, he told me to call before crossing the border, and again when coming home. We met our Amor representative at the border to Mexico and were quickly led to our campsite. That night, we said Mass around a campfire, and shared our first meal while learning of our destination.

We were assigned to build a home in a tiny village about an hour from the border. The house would be smaller than my bedroom at the rectory of St. Charles, and would be home to a family of three.

Obviously, they were extremely excited to move into a home and off
the streets.

The drive into the village was a monumental shock for
everyone, including me. It was a dunghill. It was literally built on the
side of a garbage dump, and the blistering heat created a nauseating
stench that nearly brought tears to my eyes. Completing the picture
were the wild dogs with open wounds and sores, and no electricity
or running water. Also missing was a public bathroom, so the
residents would take a bucket and head towards the dump to take
care of business.

Charlie's Angels were speechless.

So were the adult chaperones.

So was the priest.

It was beyond shocking. We couldn't believe that just twenty-
four hours earlier, we woke up and showered with hot, running
water, and spent the rest of the time choosing appropriate attire for a
mission trip while nursing a healthy breakfast.

We worked from 8:00AM to 5:00 PM, but the experience went
far beyond building a home. The kids, with chaperones, had time to
stroll down the streets in groups and meet with other families in the
neighborhood. One of the things we quickly noticed was that in a
world devoid of cable TV and other assorted gadgets of comfort, the
most precious blessing the people had was each other. Our
youngsters watched intently as mothers held their children and sang
to them. The Angels were astonished to see the same mothers
offering whatever food they had, and how the men never came home
from work without pausing to kick a soccer ball around with his son
or daughter. Our kids never said a word, but I could tell they were
taking in every moment.

I was deeply moved as well. The Jesus of my youth was alive
and well on these streets; I could feel His presence in the midst of dire
poverty, and so could our kids. Each night when we finished work,
we would gather outside the tiny house, and people throughout the
neighborhood would join us for prayer. Although I didn't speak
Spanish, many of our kids did, so we offered a combined

English/Spanish prayer to our Lord that was simply beautiful. I found myself quietly slipping away more than once to contain my emotions.

The second day at our work site, I got sick—again. It was always the same pattern; I would begin by losing my voice, and then develop a cold, which would slip down my chest and land in my lungs. Although I brought medications with me, we actually had to send a van load of people into a nearby village in search of cough medicine. I was starting to get frustrated as one cold and infection followed another. I couldn't shake it, and I began to wonder if it could be heart related. The thought was fleeting, and I decided I was too young for such problems, and just needed some rest.

It was quite a scene the afternoon we pounded in the last nail, and the family began moving their belongings into the little home. There wasn't a dry eye among us. We gathered in a circle and prayed together for the last time, ending with the family thanking us for our efforts. In turn, we thanked them for allowing us into their lives

Driving back to our campsite, one of the Angels offered a beautiful reflection. "I came down here feeling sorry for the people," she said, "but over the last few days I watched how they held their children and talked to them for hours. I watched how they offered us what little they had. I don't know if they would like some of my life, but I would love some of theirs."

This came from a teenager who received a car for her 16th birthday.

The youngsters saw through the poverty to the quality of the families' love. They were so moved that many later spoke publically on what they learned. They witnessed love that couldn't be bought, and it was alive even in the direst of conditions. It forced us to consider our own lives back home.

We returned to our campsite for a dinner of burgers and hot dogs, and offered Mass for the last time in Mexico. Once again, the youngsters were very emotional as they shared in the homily and relived the feelings and emotions that had been building throughout the week.

All these years later, the first Mexico mission trip with Charlie's Angels remains one of the most spiritual experiences of my priesthood. It was the simplicity that touched me; there was nothing fancy about our prayer or worship, but it was so real and heartfelt. Living in a tent for a week had its moments, but it also felt like being on a retreat, and it was beautiful to pray and center myself in God's care under an open sky.

The evenings were windy and cold, so I'd snuggle into a sweatshirt and jacket and lose myself in praying The Office (the daily prayer a priest offers twice a day) while listening to the wind blow and coyotes howling in the far distance. It was beautiful.

When you live in a world of drugs and alcohol, life gets very complicated. I spent so much time setting up deals, planning deals, and covering up my lies, that life was exhausting. Nothing was simple, and everything was complex with hidden issues and agendas. So when I experience something that is wonderful and beautiful in its simplicity, I really treasure the moment. And that is what I will always remember about the trip—no drug, chemical, or quick high could touch the feeling of working alongside dedicated people and sharing quality time in community.

When we arrived home, many of our parishioner's were there to greet us. The kids were filled with stories and shared with anyone who would listen. In the weeks that followed, I received phone calls from several neighboring parishes and churches throughout the Archdiocese wanting to know how to organize a similar trip for their students.

In the years to follow, Charlie's Angels grew and grew. The mission trip became part of the yearly routine sponsored by the parish. The last I heard, over fifty people went on the most recent mission, and I am delighted and proud of the community for supporting the youth with a powerful experience of faith.

26

Suicide — Darkness of Loss

On the road home, we pulled off the highway for some rest and a chance to stretch and I used the opportunity to call home and share the good news of our successful mission with Mom. I could tell something was wrong from the sad tone of her voice.

Gently, she explained that my young cousin had taken her life the previous evening. While I was far away celebrating Mass at the campsite, she walked into her bedroom, sat on at the edge of her bed, pulled a small pistol from her dresser drawer and shot herself.

I remember standing at the phone booth unable to speak. The week before we left for Mexico I had bumped into her at a local coffee shop. Our brief conversation was light and just small talk. We asked about our families, wished each other a relaxing break for summer, and that was it. The conversation was nothing. And now, barely into her twenties, she was dead...by her own hand.

Loss strikes again.

I didn't know her well, but I'd always enjoyed her company at family gatherings. Silly laughter coupled with a witty sense of humor, she was fun to be around. There was a tangible sweetness about her and a quiet sensitivity that made me sit up and listen when she spoke. Mom asked that I call my aunt as soon as we arrived home to help with the funeral arrangements. I would offer the homily.

I sought a quiet moment away from the Charlie's Angels kids to allow the shock and sorrow to sink in. Like anyone who has lost a family member to suicide, I was numb with disbelief. She was so kind-hearted. How could she do this to herself? I helplessly wondered about the pain and despair she must have been feeling those last days, weeks, months…years? How could I have missed it the last time we spoke?

I sat for a few moments of prayer and asked Jesus of the Cross, the Jesus who knew suffering and helped save me from my addictions, to be with my aunt and extended family during such unspeakable grief. I had no doubt that my cousin was now resting peacefully in Jesus' arms. I also knew that He would comfort her with love and understanding. I knew it because I had experienced it during my own struggle for sobriety.

It was surreal driving the last miles home with a van full of happy teens when my own cousin—not much older than the Angels—was gone. I had never offered a Mass where the deceased had taken their own life, and I had no idea what to say or even how to begin.

The morning of the funeral Mass, I woke up before dawn and offered my typical morning prayer. I thanked God for the gift and blessing of my sobriety, and humbly asked that He keep me on the right path during the day. I wondered what Jesus would say to my young cousin, and I decided that He would shower her with love by wrapping His arms around her and taking her home to rest. He would take her off the path she'd led and bring her to His place of safety. After all, Jesus had done that for me in this life, so I had no doubt He would do it for her in the next.

During the homily, I mentioned that many of us might be wondering where has our young cousin, daughter, sister, and friend gone. It's my belief that she's gone no further than God, the Good Shepherd who will leave the ninety-nine who have it all together, and go off in search for the one who is lost. That is our prayer and that is our faith. I believe he found my cousin and brought her home.

I learned an important spiritual lesson from my poor cousin: I need to constantly be vigilant in my prayer and spirituality and, as a priest, I need to be more aware of the pain of others. I need to slow down and take more time to listen where they are. To this day, it bothers me that our last meeting was so short and meaningless. If I knew that was the last time I would ever see her, I would have shared more time—who knows, maybe I would have sensed the darkness of her struggle.

I know what it's like when you think all is lost and there's no hope of reconciliation. I felt it with Steve's death, and I felt it when I couldn't stop myself from using my first year in the seminary. I have looked into the same hole my cousin did, and that is why I could never judge her actions. Only God knew the depth of her pain and her utter frustration to climb out of it.

It was pure grace that allowed me to find my way back while she continued to suffer. I hit bottom while in the seminary and I had people who were there to help, while she found herself alone. Rest in peace, young cousin, you are now with God.

Her death underscored the importance of our work with Charlie's Angels—if nothing else, the kids had people they could turn to in their moment of doubt and sorrow. It became a new and wonderful ministry in the parish.

27

Vocation Director and Archbishop Levada

How do you know when you are following God's will? How can you say for sure that you are actually following His call?

When I speak at parish events or school functions, I always say that following God's will is the key for me to remain clean and sober, but how do I know I'm actually doing it? How can I be sure that I'm keeping my own desires and pride out of it?

I think it is rooted within our prayer. For me, prayer is always more effective when I am *listening* as opposed to rambling on with chatter. When I listen, I allow myself more time to *feel*, to have a deeper sense of God's presence when I'm quiet and still. But even then, I sometimes fool myself. I know 'm heading for trouble when my own ego gets in the way and tries to take over.

The key, at least for me, is slipping into deep, solitary, contemplative prayer; the kind of prayer where I just listen to God's spirit and seek where it is leading me. I can't afford to clutter it with other thoughts. I just need to sit still and listen, and open my heart to His call, and then pray for the courage to move on it.

Not long after our mission trip, I received a call from the Office of Archbishop Levada. His secretary announced that the Archbishop wanted to see me the following afternoon. I explained that I couldn't make it because I was going to a Giants baseball game the next day. She replied that the Archbishop was looking forward to seeing me at noon the following afternoon. Yep, I missed the game.

Although I was due for a transfer within the next year or so, I had no idea what to expect. Just to cover my bases, I began reviewing previous homilies to see if I'd said anything that might upset the Archbishop. Had I butchered a contemporary theological teaching, or had I unknowingly offended anyone with a quip or wise remark at Mass? It's always a possibility.

I had a rather tense relationship with the Archbishop. I always thought he respected my passion and energy, but was wary of my judgment. I think he saw me as immature and prone to missing the bigger picture of issues related to Church.

Archbishop Levada was the only person in the entire Archdiocese of San Francisco who did *not* approve of Charlie's Angels working alongside Amor Ministry in Mexico, and was upset that I hadn't sought formal written permission from the Bishops in Mexico regarding our work with a non-Catholic group. Honestly, I'd never given it a thought.

However, the Archbishop was concerned that the people of Amor Ministry, along with other faith-based youth groups, might proselytize our kids during the trip. That raised an interesting question since I (embarrassingly) didn't know what proselytize meant. But I figured it had to mean something like pulling our kids over to the other side. It reminded me of tales my Dad told me about scarf attire at local soccer games—his point being to never mingle with "the other side."

From the Archbishop's perspective, it showed a lack of planning and protocol on my part in not getting their permission. From my perspective, I thought the Bishops had more pressing matters to worry about than teenagers working alongside groups of other faiths building homes for the poor in Mexico.

For the life of me, I couldn't understand his concern. During this time, the Archdiocese of San Francisco was suffering, as more than one highly respected Monsignor was being carted off in handcuffs to face abuse charges—and he was worried about a bunch of kids building homes for poor people because they dared share campsites with people of other faith traditions? If the concern hadn't been brought to me, I never would have believed it.

With that as our background, I was a tad nervous about our hastily called meeting the following afternoon. Deep down, I was prepared for a lecture of some sort.

But the next day, the Archbishop greeted me warmly and welcomed me into his private office. Nope, we were not there to discuss the woeful hitting slump of the Giants or building homes for the poor in Mexico. Instead, he expressed his desire for me to serve as Vocation Director for the Archdiocese. I was stunned. No, I was way past stunned—I was speechless; absolutely flabbergasted. I figured I had to be the least likely candidate in the entire priesthood he would choose for such a position. But from the beginning, it was very clear that he was serious about the offer.

The Archbishop recognized the serious shortage of priests, along with a steadily declining enrollment at St. Patrick's Seminary, and he wanted me to organize parish vocation groups and do more outreach to potential seminarians. Furthermore, he wanted me to speak at parishes, high schools, and colleges on the joys and blessings of serving the church as a priest.

The role of Vocation Director is very important because he or she (it is almost always a priest) works closely with the local Bishop and the seminary staff in evaluating future seminarians and priests. I thought it said a lot about the Archbishop that he was willing to appoint me for the job, despite our recent disagreement.

I asked for a night to think and pray about it, and he agreed. However, while walking me to the door, he reinforced his desire; "I want you for this job."

When I arrived home at St. Charles, I went immediately to the Church and sat down for some serious prayer. In my heart of hearts, I knew I wasn't the type to work in the Chancery Office for the Archbishop. God bless those who can do it, but there is no way it's for me. I knew it. God knew it. My family knew it. All my friends knew it. Fr. Ryan knew it. It was quite clear—I am just not the right person for such a job. I'm not the office type. The idea of being out in the community was attractive, but taken as a whole, it simply was not a good fit for my personality.

I sat in the church pew and opened my heart to God's will; "Lord, I will do whatever You want, just please give me some direction."

In prayer, I was convinced that the Good Lord was warning me not to accept the position and stay with what I do best, which is working in parish and school communities. As Fr. Bob Gavin told me when I first entered the seminary, "God brought you here to share your story in the hopes of helping others in similar situations."

In the end, there was no doubt in my mind that God was calling me to let go of my ambitions and settle back into the work I was doing at St. Charles. And while I was convinced that the right and proper response was to thank the Archbishop and return to the parish, the old, ever-present ego got in the damn way again. Somehow, I began to think that working in such a position might validate my comeback from drinking and using in my twenties. It would be like telling myself, "OK, you made it all the way back. Congratulations. Way to go, Joe."

In an instant my sense of God's will vanished only to be taken over by my highly developed ego and sense that *I* knew better, even though every time I followed such a path, it led to unmitigated disaster.

To this day it amazes me the depth and power of my need to control the path I will take. Oh, I will *say* it's God's will, and maybe even mean it, but if it is something I desire, I will still push for it, which, in turn, causes my own demise. Amazing.

I took the time and spoke with close friends in the priesthood, and to a person, they felt the image of me working out of a desk in the Chancery Office was flat out comical, worthy of a hilarious skit at the next seminary talent show.

So, against the advice of everyone who cared about me, and against the sense I had of God's will, I walked into the kitchen of the rectory, found Fr. Ryan, and foolishly announced I would accept the position and do everything I could to raise vocation awareness throughout the Archdiocese. I would be a damn hero to myself.

My decision had nothing to do with assisting seminarians or working with newly ordained priests; it had everything to do with self-justification. It was completely rooted in Pride and Ego…the two biggest factors that have always led me into trouble.

Several weeks later, I started my new prestigious job. I arrived at the office at 9:00AM and knew I had made a terrible mistake by 9:15AM. It took all of fifteen minutes to ask myself, "What have I done?" Yep, once again I moved God's will to the background and disregarded advice from knowledgeable people in order to allow my own prideful desires rule the day. And once again, I would pay for it.

The Big Book of A.A. makes it abundantly clear that most of our difficulties and challenges stem from our ego run amok. It was hard to deny that I was a walking, breathing, living example of the accuracy of that statement. More to the point, I was angry and disappointed in myself.

I immediately missed parish life; I missed the hustle and bustle of daily life in a large community. I missed the house calls and working with all the various clubs and committees associated with a large, active parish.

As Vocation Director, I struggled with the interviews and recommendations for potential seminarians. With my own background of drinking, using, dealing, and stealing forever etched in my mind, it was difficult to look at an eager applicant and explain that he was not qualified to enter the seminary.

Who was I to turn *anyone* away? I felt unworthy to evaluate and judge the qualifications of men applying to become a priest. The seminary was pivotal life-changing moment for me. It's where I got sober and where I came to understand myself and my God much better. I grew more in my seven years of seminary training than at any other time in my life. I owed it my life.

I remember interviewing a potential seminarian who had a background eerily similar to mine; he had been to hell and back but actually had quality sobriety behind him. Nonetheless, his local pastor didn't feel he was ready for the seminary and refused to offer a recommendation. It was up to me to explain to the man that, after completing the process of applying, he was not accepted into the seminary. I had to do this while knowing full well that I was still using the entire first year at St. Joseph's. I couldn't look at myself in the mirror after such a heartbreaking discussion with a very hurt applicant. The look on his face haunted me, and it was so clear that I was not the right person for the job.

With some additional prayer, which I should have done before accepting the role as Vocation Director, I made the decision to leave. I hung around for a year, then submitted my resignation. Archbishop Levada accepted it and replaced me within twenty-four hours. I know he was disappointed in me, and he had every right to be. I promised myself to never let my ego get the best of me again…it is way too dangerous.

28

Return to Serra

The average term for service as a Vocation Director is about eight to ten years, so I'd set something of a record for shortest term in recent history. Obviously, in the closed, insulated world of the clergy, it became a newsworthy item. The word went out among the fellas that I quit too soon and never really gave it a chance. More than one pastor took the time to call me and explain the errors of my ways. Not much I could say, since I deserved it. The priests were right. I owed it to them, the Archbishop, and the seminarians to give it a real chance. No doubt I acted too quickly and should have given it more time. I think it was an example of the immaturity the Archbishop was concerned about, and I knew I'd let a lot of people down by walking away so quickly.

However, there was another side to it. No one, including myself knew just how bad my heart was. No one knew that I was walking around with dilated cardiomyopathy and my heart could give out at any moment. No one knew that I drank four, sometimes five cups of coffee a day for energy, and the fact that the hot coffee was great for breaking up my nonstop cough. No one knew because I never said anything. No one knew what I was dealing with, so they just assumed I quit on them.

Nonetheless, the Archbishop put all feelings aside and assigned me to a place where he knew I would thrive. He reassigned me to my alma mater, Serra High School, to teach and serve in Campus Ministry. In addition, he assigned me to St. Catherine's, where I grew up as a child.

The Archbishop was sending me home and allowing me to teach in a classroom.

I was assigned by the administrators at Serra to teach an upper division class and to help on various retreats throughout the year. The class was called, "Christology," which was a look at the human and divine Jesus through the four Gospels. In addition, I also taught a class on Church History.

I loved every minute of it. I felt that, once again, Divine Providence had been remarkably good to me. The first day of class, I stood before my students in full clerical attire and delivered the following address by way of introduction:

"Fellas, this class isn't an easy bullshit A. This is about life and death. There is something at stake here, and I want you fully engaged in our discussions. In my classroom, I want you to think for yourselves. You don't have to agree with me, but I want you to explain why you support the beliefs you do. We are going to examine how this Jewish carpenter challenges our opinions and decisions, and how he impacts our lives.

"I have been around, my young brothers, and have made many mistakes—I drank, used drugs, cheated, and stole from unsuspecting people who had the nerve to trust me. I believe my irresponsible actions led to the death of a dear friend…and we'll talk about that. I have watched myself become saved from myself. This Jesus who suffered and died for us literally stepped in and saved my life. He still saves it every day I'm alive and clean…and we'll talk about that, too. So, my brothers, this class is one you will remember for a long time. Let's begin."

For better or worse, I wanted to grab their attention from the first moment we met, and never let go. I didn't want them to make the same mistakes I had or walk around with the same regrets. I wanted to light a fire so they could see that this class, our class, would genuinely impact their lives. I believed God had saved me and brought me into his priesthood to do this kind of work, and I was profoundly grateful to the Archbishop for the assignment.

I wanted to give my students a foundation of faith rooted in rock, not sand, as it had been in my early life. I hoped they would see something in the Jesus of the Cross that spoke intimately to their own struggles of growing up in a fast-paced, complex culture and society.

Sound too preachy? Maybe. Well, probably.

Each morning when I arrived at school, I would immediately head to the chapel and read the daily prayer from my small twenty-four-hour book on sobriety, a book that offers practical thoughts and prayers for the former user to consider. There, I would ask God to guide me throughout the day and help me to be a positive influence on my students. I was no longer seeking personal tributes or pats on the back, I was simply there to serve and hopefully inspire them to see the joy and blessing of a faith-filled life. I wanted them to open their hearts to God's word, so when they ran into difficult and challenging times, they wouldn't run away and use as I had.

I shared my story as a testimony to God's love and mercy, and my message was always the same; "Fellas, it's way hard out there in the world, and you need someone more powerful than yourself to believe in. You'll need a sense of community to trust to get through the challenges coming your way. Trust me, guys, without the grace of God and a compassionate community, I probably would still be out there playing the same silly games and finding myself on the fringe of more trouble."

I think the boys appreciated my honesty…I know their parents did.

But while I absolutely loved my work, I found myself running out of energy. I noticed that as the year progressed it became more and more difficult to climb a single flight of stairs. I'd get about half way up and would have to pause for air. At a certain point, I simply started using the elevator just to get to the second floor.

As usual, I pretended everything was fine and ignored the symptoms by going about my work. I knew there was something wrong — most likely with my heart — and I knew I needed to see a doctor, but I kept putting off making the call. Ironically, after avoiding the obvious in my own life, I would enter my classroom and ferociously inspire the kids to never "hide from their problems."

This went on for a few years. I would have days when my energy was really good and others when I could barely get up for school in the morning. I was constantly losing my voice and had a nagging cough that just wouldn't quit.

One day I actually did break down and call a doctor who confirmed what I'd been told previously by my primary doctor—I had adult asthma. So I went on a steroid treatment program and every inhaler known to Man, and received some temporary relief. But I knew it was something more. I knew it was my heart.

After several years in the classroom, I received an unexpected call from Archbishop Levada. I cringed when I received notice that I was to schedule an appointment with him as soon as possible. As usual, I had no idea what to expect.

Once again, the Archbishop caught me off guard by informing me I was to serve as President of Serra High School. After my short and disappointing performance as Vocation Director, I figured my days of serving in a high profile position were long gone. And because of that, I didn't apply for or seek the job. Instead, I was handed the assignment.

I admit to being a better teacher than administrator. My heart will always be in the classroom; it's where I'm energized to offer my best. I loved planning lessons and having discussions with my students on the moral issues of the day.

Although I was blessed to receive wonderful support from faculty and staff, I soon began to wear down under the nonstop pace of administrative work. The long, late-night meetings began to take their toll almost immediately. My cough got worse, and there were days I sat in my office, too afraid to physically exert much energy. It was starting to get scary as my heart seemed to pound so rapidly in my chest that I would frequently break out in a sweat.

One afternoon while offering a presentation on future enrollment at the school, my heart temporarily stopped beating. I mean, it actually missed more than one beat, leaving me pale with sweat dripping down my brow. It was like being on a roller coaster. First, my heart would feel like it was flying out of my chest, and then it would suddenly slow down to the point where it began to miss a beat. It was terrifying.

I asked to be excused for a moment from the presentation and walked to the nearest restroom where I sat until it passed. I remember looking at my face in the mirror and being shocked as it was completely flushed and covered with sweat. I knew I was in trouble.

No doubt, I should have called 911 and waited for an ambulance, but instead, I decided to wait it out, wipe the sweat off my face, and return to the meeting. From that day on, I would drop a few aspirin into my pocket each morning and eat one or two when I felt my heart get tight or begin to beat rapidly.

I was remarkably stupid for not seeking professional help. The main problem was that there was never any time to prepare for one of the episodes. It would literally come out of nowhere. I could be standing or sitting, walking, or even resting in bed, and it would start. I would try and relax and pray for it to stop, but I could no longer deny that there was a serious problem.

As my energy waned, I started to miss classes and meetings, and even called to reschedule mass—something I had never done at any time in my priesthood. There was no doubt I was heading for something catastrophic. My physical health was also affecting my spiritual health as well; I just didn't have the drive or passion I once had. The simple act of walking took so much out of me that I didn't have the energy for school.

I could hear rumors about my health and well-being echoing from the faculty and even the kids. "Fr. Joe has lost his drive," or "Fr. Joe just doesn't seem to have the same spirit as before," or, as a faculty friend once said while cornering me after another episode, "What the hell is going on with you? You seem to be fading out on us."

I was planning on taking some time to undergo a battery of tests with a cardiologist, when one afternoon my sister called to say that

Mom had taken ill and was on her way to the hospital. When I arrived, it was obvious that Mom was more than sick; she was in the process of dying. Her heart had begun to fail and it was causing major problems with other organs.

I didn't want to waste whatever precious time I had left with Mom so, once again, I put off meeting with a doctor. The cardiologist could wait; I wanted as much time with Mom as possible.

We were blessed to spend the next few weeks with her as she fought the good fight for life. One night near the end of her struggle, I asked how she was feeling. "I'm just waiting, I had communion this morning, so I'm fine." Then, she seemed to perk up and said, "Joe, last night I woke up and felt a presence in the room. I have no doubt it was your Dad—he was here. He was standing next to me by the bed just waiting to take me home."

Mom looked so serene when she said it. I couldn't hold back the tears. In the end, I had the opportunity to thank her for the love and support she gave me throughout my life. I'm so glad I had the chance to offer an apology for the challenging times I gave her while growing up. I'm grateful that I was able to look into her eyes and tell her I loved her and would miss her, but I knew she would be safe with God and Dad. She appeared so content that it helped calm me. In fact, she even took the time to tell me what she wanted for her funeral Mass, and concluded with a gentle reminder to "keep the homily short."

I was blessed to offer Mom's funeral Mass and even gave the homily, although I'm afraid it wasn't as short as she would have liked. Maureen and Johnny helped prepare the liturgy, and we were surrounded by the love of family and friends. I publically thanked Mom for teaching us the ways of faith. I think a mother's love is very Christ-like. It is gentle and forgiving; it is unyielding and encouraging. To me, it speaks to us about Jesus. We celebrated Mom's life as best we could, and honored her new life—at home, and at peace with God and Dad.

29

Leave of Absence From the Priesthood

After Mom's passing, I returned to school, where the episodes of heart trouble increased. I spoke with the principal of Serra, Lars Lund, and informed him that I was done. I simply didn't have the physical energy to continue and was going to seek an appointment with the Archbishop and ask for a leave of absence. Lars and the faculty were stunned, but I felt it was the right and proper decision. I didn't belong in the role of president if I couldn't offer my best.

Even my homilies suffered. Bluntly put, they were terrible and delivered with half-assed intensity. I had always prided myself on rocking the house when I preached, but I didn't have the energy or spirit to deliver. Even the kids sensed something was wrong. "Hey, what's up with Fr. Joe? That homily sucked." They were right. I didn't put the time in to prepare it properly and robbed them of the opportunity to be inspired by the Gospel.

I wondered if the lack of energy was due to grief at the loss of Mom, given that this was my first time grieving "raw," without the aid of alcohol and drugs to soothe my spirit and calm my emotions. This time, I was determined to allow myself to feel exactly what was going on. When you are used to hiding your emotions in a bottle or vial, it takes a little time to adjust. But this time, I didn't want to hide. I wanted to *feel*.

There was the fear that I was losing my vocation. I had no energy or enthusiasm for anything. I'd finally reached the point where my health was an issue, and I could no longer pretend it would just go away. Nope, this one was here to stay.

I called the Archbishop and asked for a meeting. This time, it was the Archbishop who didn't know what to expect. Within the week, I met with Archbishop Levada and Auxiliary Bishop John Wester and explained that I needed a leave of absence from my life as a priest. I had no idea how long, but it might be a very long time. I honestly didn't know.

Immediately, the Archbishop sat up with concern and asked, "What's wrong?"

I told that I just didn't have it physically, emotionally, and spiritually, and lacked the energy to continue. I finished by telling them of my concern about my heart.

At first, both Bishops were silent. The Archbishop broke it by asking, "As your Archbishop, I need you to be honest and tell me if there is something I need to know. If there is something going on in your life, now is the time to tell me."

I was lost in thought, and didn't quite understand what he was saying.

So, he made it clear, "Is there a woman in your life?"

"No, it's nothing like that."

"Is there a problem with alcohol or drugs?"

"No."

"Is there any relationship we need to discuss?"

I knew he was referring to underage relationships; it was sad, even pathetic to bring it up, but I knew the Archbishop was doing what he needed to do.

"No, nothing like that at all."

"Then what is it? You are not feeling well? You are tired? What is going on? What is causing this? You have an assignment you love, you are doing good work, and your brother priests respect you...Are you sure there is nothing else going on?"

"No, there is nothing going on, I just can't do it anymore...at least for now."

Then, in a very measured voice, the Archbishop said, "Are you asking to leave your life as a priest? "

"Archbishop, I don't know. I just know that my heartbeat flies all over the place, and it has me concerned. For the last few years, I've had a rapid decline in energy which is not like me. I need to look at what is going on physically and how it has affected me spiritually. I just can't serve right now; I don't have it in me. That is all I can honestly tell you. There are no secrets—I just want to find out what is going on with my body and spirit. I honestly don't know what else to say because I'm at a loss myself."

With that, both Bishops promised their support. They encouraged me *not* to resign as a priest, but to accept a leave of absence. The Archbishop walked me to the door and told me to keep in touch. They were both gracious and offered to help me get settled after leaving my position at Serra. Before stepping into the hallway, Bishop Wester reached into his pocket and handed me his personal cell phone number. "I am here for you, Joe, call me anytime and we'll talk."

I didn't realize it that afternoon, but Bishop Wester was to become a major figure in my life and my family's as well.

30

Dilated Cardiomyopathy

I sat alone in my car for a long time after our meeting. My leave was granted, but I wasn't sure how to feel about it. I knew that my performance at Serra had dramatically fallen off in the past two years, and I didn't feel that my priesthood was safe and secure. Instead, I felt drained and had nothing left. It was more than burnout—I felt absolutely empty and didn't have the physical energy to continue.

I prayed and asked for God's help, but couldn't feel the old spirit and drive. I wondered if I'd fallen into a depression or if my heart was really as bad as it felt. I thought maybe I'm just not tough enough to work through the challenge of facing serious illness while working a high profile job.

Thanks to the grace of God and the loving support of my family and friends in recovery, I never considered drinking or using. I considered it a gift to remain sober while working out my health issues. But that didn't mean there weren't personal challenges.

The world of a diocesan priest is very small. Nothing is a secret; nothing is kept under the table for long. It's like living in a small town where everyone knows, or thinks they know, everyone else's business. Thus, by the time I walked out of the Chancery Office and entered my car, the word of my leave was already making the rounds of parishes throughout the Archdiocese of San Francisco. It's amazing how fast bad news flies throughout the community. The local clergy didn't like what they were hearing and, for a variety of reasons, they were quite angry with me.

When a priest takes a leave of absence, it is *always* assumed by the local clergy that something has gone terribly wrong. Priests will call their buddies and huddle around the day room TV at 5:00 PM, to catch footage of the "leave taker" on his media-sponsored "perp walk." Heck, half of the lads are eagerly anticipating it because it will be marvelous fire for the clerical gossip factory machine.

Nothing good is ever connected with a leave of absence, and each priest calls members of his tribe and tries to guess what happened, and why the priest has asked to leave his assignment. Everyone has an opinion, and everyone has a solution. The fact that none of them actually knows the person seeking the leave is completely irrelevant...it's the opinion that counts.

There are no exceptions. Whether you're a Bishop or high school president, the fact that you are seeking a leave from your duties is enough to garner gossip and critique from your brother priests. The walls shake with, "I told you," echoing from the rafters of your local parish.

Of course, your local clergyman will deny this in public, and profess heartfelt support during Sunday Mass, but trust me, deep down, they are utterly convinced that the priest who requested the leave is guilty of some kind of major offense. And within twenty-four hours, the stories only get wilder and more out of control.

The word on yours truly was a three-fold possibility:

1. Poor Joe was drinking and using again.
2. Happy Joe had fallen in love with a woman in the parish.
3. Confused Joe had fallen in love with a man in the parish.

While none of the three scenarios were remotely correct, it didn't matter. It never matters. The facts aren't relevant; it's the intrigue of the story that counts. Each possible scene has its share of supporters with "inside" information. Problem is, it's usually pure fantasy, but it does liven up cocktail hour in the rectory. In the world of clergy gossip, the only thing that matters is that the story has enough promise of scandal that it keeps the clerical phone lines and text messages alive through long nights of rectory life.

And that is how *every* leave of absence is handled by the local clergy. I guarantee it.

It usually takes a few days, but eventually the stories get whittled down to a brief glimpse of reality—Fr. Joe *might* have some heart problems, and it has affected his life in such a manner that he wants some time away to deal with it. The reality can't hold a candle to the fictitious soap opera, but ultimately, the truth finds its way through the fog of speculation.

That said, it was abundantly clear that my name was mud among the local clergy. I understood. Throughout the history of Serra High School, a priest had always led the school as president, and I was the first one to resign. With the shortage of priests in the Archdiocese, I was not likely to be replaced by another priest in the role of president. A priest might be assigned as Chaplain with responsibilities for offering Mass and working with the faculty and students, but the days of having a priest serve as president were likely over.

I had just compromised the foothold of power that priests held on secondary Catholic schools for decades. Because I walked away from the job, we were now entering the clerical danger zone where decision-making offices might be held by a member of the laity, a man or, dare we consider…a woman. The fact that I was leaving for legitimate reasons of health wasn't relevant—this was about the bigger issue of power. Who wields it and who doesn't.

There was plenty of resentment among a sizable group of clergy. I accepted that I was in for a beating. Hell, I probably deserved it. After all, no one walks away from such a job without advance warning, and I didn't offer it. I just walked into the Office of the Archbishop and announced that I was finished. Again.

It was painfully similar to my leaving the Office of Vocations. To make matters worse, many of my brother priests felt I had officially confirmed myself a quitter. I understood that, too. After all, I had walked away from two sacred and prominent positions of responsibility, and I walked out on both of them in short order. While the criticism hurt, I understood where the priests were coming from. If it had been someone else, I might have jumped on the bandwagon, too.

Within days, the word was out: Joe is a quitter. Put a little pressure on him and he will fold like a house of cards. He always has, and he always will. All of this fed the growing innuendo that I was drinking again. The halls rang with, "I heard from someone they were concerned he was using." Oh yeah, it got ugly…it got ugly, real fast.

However, none of it was true. My heart was fading even faster than I thought it was. When the day came that I couldn't make it up the staircase, I knew I needed to contact a doctor and get to the bottom of what was happening. I knew it required a leave.

For support, I reached out to my private family and my communal friends in recovery; I needed to attend more meetings. I needed to participate in my own recovery during this latest crisis. I was determined to look at my health and my vocation face to face and see where it all came out in the eyes of God. If it took additional time, so be it.

My meetings put me in touch with people who intimately knew how I felt. They emphasized that while confronting heart disease and dealing with my decision to seek a leave of absence, I still needed to nurture and maintain my sobriety because it was the key to everything else. "First Things First," as the tried and true recovery mantra advises.

31

Collapse

I moved my belongings out of St. Catherine's and into Mom's house. It was eerily quiet. Everyone had grown up and moved out to raise families, and Mom was peacefully resting with Dad in Heaven. I spent the first week or so thumbing through old scrapbooks, reliving the good old days of my youth, and going to as many meetings and coffee gatherings as I could.

Eventually, I made contact with a local cardiologist and set an appointment at the first available opening. Unfortunately, I didn't make the appointment, but I did meet the doctor in the emergency room at Peninsula Hospital.

I woke up about 3:30 in the morning in a lather of sweat, with my heart feeling like it was about to explode out of my chest. It was a labored beat, and each breath was a struggle. I got out of bed and slowly made my way into the kitchen where I promptly collapsed. I was literally on the floor in a fetal position gasping for breath when I pulled myself up and crawled on all fours to the phone and called my sister, Maureen.

I don't know why I didn't directly call 911 for an ambulance, but while talking to Maureen, I started to feel my heart giving way again. My sister has always been the family speedster, and she was at Mom's house in record time. Craving fresh air, I locked the front door and walked gingerly to the street curb, where I offered a prayer of thanksgiving when I saw the lights of her car coming up the street.

She pulled up at the house, took one look at me and said, "Let's go, we don't have much time."

We made it to Peninsula Hospital in record time. My breathing was so bad that I barely made it out of the car and into the

Emergency Room. The on-call cardiologist, Dr. Robert Zipkin, was concerned that my oxygen levels had dropped into the low 90s, and the heart monitor alternated between fast and slow rhythmic beats. My chest felt like an elephant was sitting on it, and I was literally crying in pain. I was grateful for the shot of morphine to manage the pain. They also fed me Amiodorone—a drug used to treat life-threatening arrhythmias and relaxing an overactive heart. It definitely made a difference, and I quickly felt its effect, which helped to calm me down.

The docs also treated me with large doses of diuretics to reduce excess swelling. Before I knew it, I had several IV lines in place and was beginning to feel that the latest episode had passed. Dr. Zipkin believed otherwise and ordered a series of tests, including an echocardiogram, which gives doctors a good sense of the overall function of the heart muscle. I remember a nurse explaining that the "echo" would reveal exactly what was going on with my forty-eight year-old heart.

Dr. Zipkin received the test results and came to my bed to deliver the news; "Joe, I'm very concerned about your heart. It's clearly in failure, and I'm afraid you have dilated cardiomyopathy."

The words rang a bell—they were once used to describe Dad's heart. I remember looking directly at a very pale Maureen, and relieved there was no mirror to look at myself.

A short time later, I was wheeled out of my little room to an office where Dr. Zipkin was huddled over a computer. He showed me a photo of a normal heart, then he showed me a picture of mine. I was stunned. The damn thing was enormous. When compared to the normal heart on the opposite screen, it looked positively gigantic. Even I could tell there was something seriously wrong with it— looking so swollen and flabby, and not the least bit healthy.

Dr. Zipkin followed by showing me a brief video of a normal beating heart and another video of my heart from tests taken that morning, where it fought to flop around and beat when it felt like it. There was no rhythm to it. If I wasn't scared before, I was now. My heart was a mess, and Dr. Zipkin agreed with my conclusion.

Calmly, but firmly, he made it clear that we were dealing with a major, life-threatening problem, and I was going to be admitted to the hospital immediately and should plan to stay a while. The following morning, I would undergo an angioplasty procedure to see if any of the arteries were blocked. Additionally, the staff would monitor my heartbeat and oxygen level throughout the day and night.

I took a brief moment to let it all sink in before saying a brief prayer: "Lord, You have led and guided me since I asked for Your healing and forgiveness. I have surrendered my life to You, and I trust You. Please be with me now, and please be with my sister and brother and their families. Finally, Lord, please, I beg of You, give me the courage and strength to know and accept Your will."

I did not ask the Lord for a miraculous intervention. I just needed to be reminded that, spiritually, I wasn't alone, and I wanted the strength to accept my fate in the uncertain days to come. No agenda or immature threats if things didn't work out my way; I wanted to feel that I had finally developed a good spiritual center—one that would carry me forward.

Anyone who has ever spent more than a day in hospital knows the days are non-stop and eventful, but with the exception of emergencies, the evenings tend to be quiet. After visitors leave, it can be eerily subdued.

I got into a routine where my morning prayer was a quick check in with the Lord, but it was the quiet of the evening and the wee hours of the morning, where I established my main sanctuary of prayer. I grew to enjoy the silence of early morning prayer. The nurse would come in to check on me at 3:00AM, sometimes to check or replace an IV, sometimes to give me another medication. After she left, I would relax into prayerful reflection.

As always, I focused on Jesus of the Cross, the One who saved me from drinking and using. I would just sit with Him in the silence of my room and take in the quiet sounds of nurses tending to patients in nearby rooms. I even became sensitive to the smells of the room at such an hour. It spoke to me of life. As long as I could feel all that was around me, I was truly alive, and my body and spirit were still in the fight for life.

The ritual of prayer helped re-center me at times when my emotions threatened to take over. One early morning, Dr. Zipkin checked in to see how I was doing. I used the unexpected visit as an opportunity to thank him for his care and willingness to reach out to my family. After he completed a quick check up, I looked him in the eye. "Dr. Zipkin, I have been wondering; exactly what is the cure for dilated cardiomyopathy?"

"Unfortunately, Joe, there is no cure. Your heart is steadily declining and in failure."

He said it so calmly and empathetically that I didn't quite get what he was saying, and I paused for a long moment before continuing. "Excuse me, but did you just say that there was no cure?"

He nodded. "Let's not get a head of ourselves, ok? Let's go a day at time—there are a few more tests I want to evaluate."

I was stuck on the "no cure" part, and frankly wasn't interested in a few more tests. If my game was almost up, I wanted to know. But if there was a chance to reclaim my health, I wanted to stay in the fight. "Come on, Dr. Zipkin, surely there has to be a procedure that can fix this problem and make it work the way it used to. I mean, work with me here."

Dr. Zipkin looked at Maureen and me and asked if we had a history of heart disease in our family. Now it was my turn to laugh a little at our ridiculous family history of heart related illness. "Dr. Zipkin, my family belongs in the damn Hall of Fame for heart disease. Allow me to share some of our distinguished history. How is this for a lineup:

Dad: died at fifty-one from dilated cardiomyopathy; Aunt on Dad's side: Died at thirty-three of heart related issues and diabetes; Dad's youngest brother: Died in mid-fifties from heart related illness. Dad's middle brother: Doing great...after receiving a heart transplant at Loyola University, Illinois. The cause? Dilated cardiomyopathy.

"Let's pause, Doc, before checking out the other side of the family: Mom: Died of heart related disease; Mom's younger brother: Died of heart disease at the age of thirty-eight; Mom's older brother: Died of heart and lung disease in his sixties...his first heart attack occurred in his early forties.

"What do you think? Both sides of the family. Is that a stellar line up or what? When it comes to heart disease, the Bradley clan kicks ass."

Dr. Zipkin simply shook his head and noted, "Well, we know what we're up against. Joe, you need to know this will not be an easy or quick fix. Ultimately, the only cure for this disease is to have a heart transplant."

I'm a priest, so I will gracefully refrain from sharing my one-word response to the phrase, "Heart transplant."

I remained in hospital for two weeks. Two of my arteries were blocked, and Dr. Zipkin scheduled an additional set of exams which served to confirm his initial diagnosis.

The following months, I spent quite a bit of time as a resident of Peninsula Hospital. I had several episodes of heart failure. Dr. Zipkin tried everything, including a fairly new drug called Coreg which was supposed to help strengthen my failing heart. The combination of Coreg and Amiodarone, along with a steady diet of beta blockers and blood thinners, kept me reasonably healthy, but every few weeks I would slip into failure. There was no way of predicting when it would happen, since the disease had a mind of its own.

One afternoon, while back in hospital, Dr. Zipkin pulled up a chair near the bed and said we needed to talk. My most recent echo exam had shown my heart was continuing to decline regardless of the treatment. "Joe, I'm afraid your condition is past what we can do here at Peninsula Hospital. I believe you need to get listed for a heart transplant, and both Stanford and UCSF have excellent programs that are respected throughout the world. Choose either hospital, and I will get you an appointment with their transplant team."

I explained that I had a real problem with Stanford. It had nothing to do with their superb hospital, but it was about their football team. I loathed it. And more to the point, I had an intense dislike for their football band. Dr. Zipkin looked at me rather curiously, so I explained, "I went to a Stanford and Notre Dame football game a few years ago and the Stanford band embarrassed and insulted Notre Dame during its half time performance, and there will be no peace, love, flowers, or Kumbaya regarding such an offense. So while I wish Stanford no ill will, we will take my ailing heart to UC. It is purely a football decision, but a very important football decision."

Dr. Zipkin noted that in all his years of practicing medicine, he had never heard such an explanation, but he promised to honor it and call UC to arrange an appointment with their transplant team.

I will always cherish his care and concern...and sense of humor.

32

UCSF Medical Center: Heart and Lung Transplant Unit and Dr. Theresa DeMarco

No matter how much I prayed and tried to calm myself, I was filled with anxiety. In fact, on the drive to UCSF, I reminded Johnny that twenty-five years ago I would have asked him to stop somewhere on the way in. He laughed knowing full well what I meant. "Yeah, and by the time you finished with your 'quick stop,' we probably would have missed the appointment or blown it off completely."

I agreed. Back in the day, I could see me stopping for a quick cold one (on the way to visit a doctor about a heart transplant.) and winding up in a bar in Sausalito, drunk and sitting alone admiring the sailboats of the bay. I would have hired Keith Richards as my life coach to get through the situation.

We made our way through the maze of University of California Medical Center San Francisco, and sat down with Dr. Theresa DeMarco. When she walked into the small examination room, she couldn't help but take in the two guys who had worked themselves into a nervous lather of sweat. Her natural warmth took over as she introduced herself to us. Everything about Dr. DeMarco spoke of confidence and professionalism, and I knew I was in good hands.

I still remember her first words: "OK guys, let's just relax; we are just going to talk, so don't be scared."

Johnny and I let out a nervous laugh.

She continued, "When people step off the elevator and see the Heart and Lung Transplant Clinic sign, they often get wrapped up in fear before we have even have a chance to talk."

Dr. DeMarco was absolutely correct. We had just met, and I was half expecting her to begin carving into my chest…in the office…while chatting with friends and checking her email.

She made it clear that the journey to transplant would involve an entire team of doctors, counselors, and social workers. "The transplant community is like a big family, and we watch out for each other. You and your family will have tremendous support from throughout our community."

In five minutes Dr. DeMarco had accomplished the impossible. She put our anxieties as ease and opened the door to honest dialogue about future strategies concerning my heart. She had already reviewed all the charts and documentation sent by Dr. Zipkin, but wanted some additional testing. "Joe, I'm not going to downplay this because you have a right to know, and I will always tell you what is going on. The truth is, your heart is in very bad shape. We can do a few things to help, but in the end, we are *definitely* looking at a transplant. It's our only option to save your life."

The word that stopped me was "definitely"…as in, we are totally sure of this. I was always OK with words like "possibly" or even "likely" — but "definitely" had a whole different ring to it. There was no room for doubt, and this was now my confirmed fate.

Dr. DeMarco outlined a series of steps to begin my journey. The first was to officially get myself listed as a potential recipient of a donor heart. There were only a few more tests and a decision would be made as to whether I qualified as a transplant candidate at UCSF. If accepted, I would be registered on a national organ transplant waiting list. Then, the waiting period would officially begin.

However, before going too far into the future, Dr. DeMarco wanted to implant a pacemaker and a defibrillator in order to ease some of the discomfort from the constant bouts of heart failure. Damn. Thought for sure I was getting out of there without any cutting.

The pacemaker, along with the other drugs I had been taking since the first night in the Emergency Room, would help regulate my heartbeat. However, if my heart still slipped into failure, the defibrillator would literally kick it back into action, which meant that the defibrillator would know when my heart had missed a beat and was heading to failure, and it would shock my heart back into a normal pattern. She called it "shock therapy" — hmm, rather interesting juxtaposition of words.

I held out a small piece of hope this "shock" was nothing more than a quick, little, minor, hardly noticeable, meaningless pinprick inside my chest. "Dr. DeMarco, what exactly does 'shock therapy' feel like?"

"I'm glad you asked. People have described it as a mule kick to the chest. It can literally knock you back a step or two. It's very unpleasant, but it will literally save your life."

"Mule kick, you say? I'd hoped you might have a softer and gentler version."

"No, I'm afraid that is how it works. When missing a beat and moving to failure, your heart will need a strong shock to restart it. If the kick isn't strong enough your heart might not come back on its own, and you will die."

"Thank you, Dr. DeMarco. Let the explosions begin."

Between the medications, pacemaker, and defibrillator, Dr. DeMarco hoped to buy enough time while waiting for an available heart. That was the strategy for staying alive until my transplant.

I quickly learned that Dr. Theresa DeMarco doesn't waste time. She made plans for the surgical procedure to take place as soon as my final tests were complete. She closed the meeting with a thorough checkup, and scheduled a follow up appointment in ten days.

When she departed, a social worker came in for a chat, followed by a young intern with a clipboard full of questions. They were listed under the heading: "Lifestyle."

I squirmed a little in my seat as he began the inquisition. "Have you ever smoked tobacco?"

"No. After watching my dad die, I always had a healthy fear of it."

"Good."

"Have you ever used narcotics?"

I remember taking a long look at the floor. I felt the tension increase in the room. *Well, this ride might be over before it even begins.* I guess no matter how hard we try, our past is always with us. "Yes, I have used narcotics in the past."

"Yes?" he quietly repeated.

"Yes," I added with emphasis. "It was a lifetime ago in terms of the person I am today, but I won't lie or pretend it wasn't part of my history. I used after my dad's death; I didn't handle his loss very well. I was only twenty, but I was involved for several years."

The young intern glanced up from his writing and casually nodded, "I understand. Thank you."

And that was it. The question was never brought up or discussed again. I was obviously relieved, but I was also at peace for having faced reality and told the truth.

It was a quiet ride home. At one point, I asked Johnny if he took any notes in his spiral notebook he brought for the occasion. "No, I actually didn't write much down," he replied.

"Well, let's see what you wrote."

He slowly opened the notebook and there were only two words in the entire book: "Heart Transplant"

A little gallows humor never hurts, so we both burst into laughter. "Good job, bro, you captured the essence of the meeting."

33

Spiritual Questions and Guidance

When I arrived home from our meeting with Dr. DeMarco, I got on the computer and began researching everything I could about heart transplant surgery. The first thing I learned is it was a last resort, and a cardiologist would only recommend transplant if the patient was facing certain death and no other option was available. Dr. DeMarco said as much during our meeting.

I found several medical sites that explained and described the actual surgery. In fact, twenty minutes of research was enough for me. When I found a section entitled, "Risks of Surgery," I was quite finished. Whatever I needed to know I would learn from Dr. DeMarco and her staff. The most important thing I could do was prepare myself spiritually for what was to happen...or, to my horror, *not* happen.

I contacted Bishop John Wester and told him about my meeting with Dr. DeMarco, explaining that a heart transplant was our only option. He invited me to his private residence for lunch the following afternoon.

Bishop Wester was highly respected among the priests of the Archdiocese, and I had always held him in the highest regard. He had a wonderful presence in the community and was reliable to anyone who called on him. He was and is the epitome of what a Bishop should b —a true shepherd of his flock. John Wester lived it every day of his life.

Unlike Archbishop Levada, Bishop Wester's roots were solidly planted in parish life instead of being a Chancery Office bureaucrat, insulated from the complexities of day to day life in an active parish. To the contrary, he always had his pulse on life in the diverse parishes of the Archdiocese. I always thought that was the main reason he was so respected by the local pastors. A veteran pastor once told me, "John will be a wonderful Bishop because he has worked in the trenches and he knows the challenges of ministry at the parish level." I completely agreed with his sentiment.

When we met the following afternoon, Bishop Wester looked a bit relieved, saying, "Well, this explains your last year at Serra." I admitted my own culpability for not checking in sooner with a doctor.

After a brief lunch, we sat in his office and I shared my latest spiritual dilemma: I didn't know what to pray for. I was spiritually stuck and unable to work through it. In order to undergo a heart transplant meant that someone else had to die for me to live. I found that more difficult to accept than all the other surgeries combined. I've been capable of doing some terrible things in my life—but how can you pray for the misfortune of someone else? Of course, no one can do that.

It seems to violate everything Jesus preached and stood for. In fact, the entire Gospel message is just the opposite. Jesus modeled selfless love and sacrifice for another. The ultimate act was to lay down our life for someone else, but I was asking for the exact opposite.

Bottom line: Someone had to die so I could live.

Some poor soul had to lay down his or her life so I could regain mine. Obviously, they were not planning on it, but nonetheless *I was counting on it* to restore my own life. It was a hell of a spiritual position to be in, and I had no answer. In fact, I didn't even know where or how to start.

Looking at Bishop Wester, I said, "Ever since my ordination as a priest, I have always known what to say to someone who was sick; I even knew what to say to their families and loved ones. I packaged the message, and knew exactly how to deliver it. I was trained and taught what to say in their moment of darkness and doubt. Heck, I was good at it. I would enter a hospital room, rattle off what I had practiced, and was back in my car within the hour. I had the whole procedure down to a science. But now it is my turn. Now, I'm on the gurney and in the hospital bed. And sadly, I don't have a damn thing to say, and I don't know what to pray for. This is a humbling journey, and I've only just started."

Bishop Wester was silent for a long time. "It's different now, isn't it?"

"Hell yes, it is."

And then Bishop John Wester said something I wasn't prepared to hear: "Maybe it's time for you to do nothing."

"What, are you serious?" I leaned forward. "You mean quit? I just recently got blasted by my brother priests for being a quitter, and now you are *advising* me to quit? Come on, Bishop, what are you saying? Give me something more than 'give up.' "

He gave me a paternal smile. "You're missing the point, my friend. Maybe the time for *doing* is over, and maybe it's time to rest. I think that might be your best spiritual path. Your doctors are doing everything they can to slow down your body so it can be ready if a new heart comes your way, so maybe it's time to offer the same chance for your spirit. Let it go, my friend. Rest in God's love. Rest with Jesus. Rest in His Holy Spirit. Maybe the best way to stay in the fight is not to fight. Let God care and love you like He did in your struggle for sobriety. He is there for you, and always has been. No matter what happens, Joe, this is not a path or journey you can control anyway. There are so many unknowns, so why not just let it go completely, and let God take over."

34

Centering Prayer —
Remaining Grounded during Journey

I wanted to find a spiritual prayer form to carry me through the journey to transplant. But I didn't want to just *read* about prayer, I wanted to *experience* it on a deeper level. I suppose, like most people, I don't really pray with my head, I pray with my heart. My best prayer (if there really is such a thing) usually evolves out of my silence. When I have that kind of spiritual experience, I always walk away in a better place than when I began. It's not me making it happen, it's God's spirit. So with a test of a transplant looming ahead, I really wanted to deepen my connection with that spirit.

I have always found praying the daily Office a challenge; I love reading the Psalms and following the seasonal scripture passages, but there are times I fade out while reading. I'm not as deeply into the beautiful readings as I should be. But I remembered my study of Centering Prayer with Fr. Bob while I was still a seminarian and how it always worked for me. It calmed my emotions and helped keep my spirit grounded and at peace. I decided to read further and see if I could incorporate it into my spiritual life.

Centering Prayer might best be described as a case of "less is more;" that is, it's not what you bring to the experience that's important, it's what you don't. The key is to block everything out and simply enjoy solitary time with the Lord. I tried to consciously remove all the distractions and fears of my potential surgery, and seek nothing more than God's soothing presence. In fact, that is what I was seeking—to enter a place of "nothingness," a quiet spiritual center that is totally inhabited by God's spirit.

If I found myself wondering or feeling too edgy, I would quietly say the word "Jesus," not as a mantra, but just a quiet call to slip back into my center; the place God's spirit lived. The beauty of Centering Prayer is it requires me to live completely in the present—no looking back to joys and regrets, and no looking forward to hopes and dreams. Just now. Here. Today. This moment in time with God.

The future and the past are dangerous places for a former drunk and user to go. They are both filled with landmines that destroy recovery and kill sobriety. I need only to live in the present, and Centering Prayer helps keep me there, where I am safe and secure and know God's love.

In the year that followed, I remained true to the practice of Centering Prayer. It became my lifeline to remaining grounded as the tension of waiting for a healthy heart increased. Every morning and evening, I would slip into my own private sanctuary of spiritual nothingness, and simply allow the Lord to connect with my body and spirit. As Bishop Wester bluntly reminded me, "You have no control over this journey anyway, so why not let the Lord guide your way."

There was another humbling reality at work as I prepared myself for what transplant patients call, The Wait. The truth is, I didn't completely trust myself. I didn't trust that at some point along the path to transplant I would have a slip, and I would use again. I think the old adage is true: "Recovery isn't an end, it's a beginning." I felt I would be OK, as long as I remained humble and allowed the broken Jesus of the Cross to do for me what I couldn't do for myself.

There is a powerful passage in Matthew's Gospel (8:28-34) where Jesus enters a town and confronts and conquers two demons. When the crowd sees what happens, they are moved with fear at His power. Now, one might think they'd run to Him and embrace what He offers, but they actually beg Him to leave. They are so overwhelmed by who He is and the power He has, that they want nothing to do with him. It's almost as if they feel unworthy of His ability to heal them...so, they run away.

I understood the crowd and their reaction. I have done the same thing and felt the same way at times in my life. It was a huge hurdle for me to feel worthy of asking for His—or anyone's—help because that sense of shame was so deep. Drunks and users like me beat ourselves up all the time. We crave the high, but grow tired of using. The more we hate it, the more we lie, cheat, and steal to get it. It was like being on an endless treadmill and not being able to push the STOP button.

That's why I can relate to the people in the Gospel passage. They weren't afraid of Jesus' power to judge, but of his power to heal and restore. It was only after a few quality years of sobriety that I felt worthy to allow God and His people into my life. Trust in myself and others took time to develop. I sensed I would need both on the journey to transplant.

35

Surgery: The Defibrillator Goes Kaboom

The procedure to implant the pacemaker and defibrillator was relatively painless. I was actually discharged the following morning after the doctors monitored it during the night. However, the following night I was readmitted to UCSF when my heart slipped into deep failure. My blood pressure was 183/98, and it was a struggle to breathe. In addition, I had developed a slight fever which was now 101 degrees and slowly rising.

The roller coaster ride had officially begun.

The ride by ambulance into UC was full throttle—lights, sirens, the works. I'd broken down and called 911 when I could no longer move because my breathing had slowed to nothing, and my blood pressure kept rising. As we flew onto the freeway, I suddenly started to relax and slip into a remarkably peaceful sleep. I think I would have kept going had someone in the back of the ambulance not shouted, "Stay with me, Joe."

I don't consider it a near-death experience, but it was a very strange feeling. One minute the discomfort and struggle to breathe (even with oxygen) had me besieged and frightened, and the next minute I was completely relaxed and slipping into a lovely, tranquil state. When I came to, I heard someone say, "Just stay with me, we're almost there."

As we entered the Emergency Room (again) I told God I was ready. While being wheeled into a room, I apologized to the Lord for the mistakes in my life. I also used the opportunity to thank Him for the years of sobriety, and the love and support of my family and the larger community. If this was it, I wanted to make my peace with God. I wasn't scared; I was ready for anything.

The tests they took in the Emergency Room found that a small amount of fluid was building at the base of my heart. If that wasn't enough, I had an infection in my one of my lungs. Since I was a transplant patient, I was admitted to the Cardiac Intensive Care Unit where I remained for several days. Eventually, I was released to the 10th floor Transplant Unit, and was treated for another week. A pattern was developing where I was home for a week or so, then back in the hospital with another bout of heart failure.

After some time, I was released and allowed to go home. It felt wonderful being in our house again, and I was determined to rest and slowly make my way back to full health. After a day or two, I decided to go for a walk. As I opened the front door to walk out into the beautiful sunshine, I felt my heart pause and skip a beat or two…KABOOM. The defibrillator went off. It literally knocked me back through the door. I lay there for a few minutes to get my bearings, and as I started to get up…KABOOM…it knocked me back down again.

By this time, I was getting used to crawling across the kitchen floor to a phone. I reached up to call 911…KABOOM…the damn thing went off a third time. This one drove me across the floor, where I rolled onto my back. All told, the defibrillator went off eleven times in forty minutes.

It took forever to reach the phone because the damn thing kept exploding in my chest. Eventually, I got angry, which only heightened my blood pressure and made the heart go faster—which made it skip a beat or two—which made the defibrillator blow up again.

Eventually, I got hold of 911, and was off for yet another trip to UCSF. I was becoming a familiar figure and got to know the Emergency Room people on a first name basis. A young doctor, who looked all of fifteen, met me in the cardiac room as the nurse was preparing me for another echo exam. The doctor, an expert in the ways of defibrillator blow ups, had somehow checked on the device and confirmed that I had received eleven jolts of Shock Therapy.

"Helluva description," I grunted, the model of patience, humility, and brotherly love. How 'bout, 'Taser Ass Kick Explosive'?"

Moments later, Dr. DeMarco arrived and calmly assured me that the defibrillator had done its job…harrowing as that might be.

I was sent back to the 10th floor for yet more tests, where I learned about a certain Catch-22 involved with the angry piece of machinery called a defibrillator. While it shocks the heart into a more normal rhythm and brings it back to life, the jolt also damages the muscle. Because mine went off so often, it was doing great harm to the very organ it was trying to save. Great. What next?

As my heart continued to fade, I was told it was no longer safe for me to drive. I understood, but it was tough to lose another piece of my independence. But if my defibrillator went off again, there was no way I could control my car. Maybe I could handle one jolt, but once this baby got going, there was no stopping it. I didn't want to be responsible for injuring someone on the road, so I turned over my keys.

That was yet another lesson I learned; when people are sick, they lose much more than just their physical health. There are all sorts of complexities attached and incredible as it seems, I never really considered it when I would visit the sick in our parish. I just offered care, presided at an anointing, and left. The day I put my car keys in the dresser drawer, I promised myself to take an entirely different attitude when visiting the sick. But first, I had to get my own health back where I could see a future of working with the sick.

In an effort to reduce the swelling of my heart, we hastily scheduled surgery to siphon fluid from the base of my heart. I was released a few days later and felt much better. As I was being discharged, Dr. DeMarco reminded me that we were buying time and I should check into the Transplant Clinic the following week for additional tests to monitor the condition of my heart post-surgery. She gave me her private office number and said I, or anyone in my family, could call anytime.

36

Looking At Death

Throughout the next twelve months, I spent more time in hospital than out. I did my best to follow Bishop Wester's advice — to rest in God's love and allow the process to play itself out. Centering Prayer became my absolute salvation. What started as five minutes of prayer in the morning and evening evolved into a half-hour. I treasured the soothing feeling of knowing the spirit of the Lord was with me.

During one of the hospital stays, tests revealed an increase of fluid buildup at the base of my heart. It explained the constant gurgling sound I could hear when I lay down or took a deep breath. Dr. DeMarco advised surgery to drain the excess fluid. It was a major procedure called a Pericardial Window, where the surgeon makes an incision in my chest and inserts a hose to siphon out the excess fluid that was smothering my heart and making it work even harder.

Dr. Theresa DeMarco wasn't a person to mince words, and she told me that one of these times my heart would go into failure and, even though the defibrillator would shock it back, my heart would slip again until one day when it wouldn't come back. While the surgery was serious and viewed as a last resort that was fraught with risks, it was still a stopgap measure to buy some time while waiting for a transplant.

Dr. D put her hand on my shoulder and said, "Joe, time is not our friend. We will do everything we can, but you have a right to know where we are. No one is giving up, but your heart isn't doing well and continues to swell, and I know you are very uncomfortable."

I nodded and paused to consider my own death.

That night after my brother and sister went home, I wrote out the plans for my funeral Mass. Surprisingly, it wasn't as emotional an experience as I thought it would be. I felt more pragmatic. Facts were that if I didn't receive a new heart soon, my time was limited. Maybe a month, maybe less; I could literally feel my body slipping away.

I asked that Bishop Wester serve as the Main Celebrant of the Mass, and John Ryan, who taught me so much about ministry during my early years serving at St. Charles Parish, would offer the homily. It seemed right. Bishop Wester had been remarkably generous with his time, and his weekly visits meant so much to my family and me.

I also asked that a priest who helped me immensely my first years of sobriety offer the final prayers of commendation. Remaining sober had been the greatest blessing of my life; it was living proof that God has the power to heal and restore. Lastly, I made a special request that my funeral be a celebration of life. So many people had stood by me in the darkness, so I wanted the Mass to be uplifting and hopeful. I believe that with faith in God and faith in His people, there is always hope.

I chose "Be Not Afraid," as the Entrance Hymn because I wasn't afraid of anything anymore. It was also the opening hymn of my ordination Mass, so I thought it would be entirely appropriate to offer it at my funeral Mass.

I requested a special hymn for the recessional song, "Blue Sky," by the Allman Brothers Band. Oh yeah, I thought it might be spiritually uplifting to listen to some beautiful, melodic guitar on my way out of the church.

And while I wanted to leave a message of hope, I wasn't ready to give up on the life I was blessed to have. I wanted to live. But obviously it was out of my hands. Of course, the sad irony is if I was visiting a patient who was facing possible death while waiting for a transplant, I knew what I would say to him or her.

I would encourage them to pray and make peace with God and their family, and ask for the strength to accept God's will. I would also assure them that the good Lord was with them through their struggle, and then I would offer communion before making my way to the door. But somehow, such priceless pastoral advice wasn't working as well when I offered to myself. Why? Because, damn all, I wanted to live.

I remember reading a quote attributed to Cardinal Joseph Bernadine during the last years of his battle with cancer when he was looking at his own death. I had always admired his courage and gentle pastoral presence. He was a bishop and, ultimately, a Cardinal, and despite his clerical success, he never lost touch with his people. As he considered his impending death, he noted that the key to maintaining a sense of peace was twofold:

1. He believed that he must place himself completely in the hands of God with absolute trust.
2. He began to see death not as an enemy but as a friend.

I understood his first point because it was the key to my sobriety and recovery. Left to my own design and will, my life became completely unmanageable. I lost control over my using and fell into a deep abyss to the point where I couldn't begin to even contemplate a way out.

However, the Cardinal's second point threw me for a loop. I mean I never, *ever* considered looking at death as a friend. Perhaps, a worthy foe to fight, but *not* a friend. I wasn't ready to give in to heart disease.

But when I carefully considered the depth of Cardinal Bernadine's spirituality, I could see and even understand his point. Death was our natural end, but it was also our new beginning. It was the moment we would meet God face to face. It was actually the ultimate vision of safety because we were finally and eternally home. If I looked at it that way, it was actually rather soothing…like a friend. There was nothing to fear if it meant returning to a loving, healing, forgiving God who promised eternal life.

It seemed like I often walked right to the edge, right to the point where I was ready to completely abandon myself to God, but I always held back a little, and that definitely impacted my attitude towards death. I knew that the Cardinal was advocating a complete willingness to let go of *everything*—even Life itself. I think it was more than a statement of trust; it was a statement of deep love.

Even in sobriety, I always seemed to keep a tiny spot for myself. It was a like a secret room where I could wander; I think it's why I always considered my sobriety such a grace because I believe God brought me back from the brink, into His presence, His home, even when I still held back. I believe that's why the Cardinal considered death a friend—not that he wanted it—but he recognized our death was just a new beginning of an even deeper relationship with God. I'm not sure if I ever arrived at the spiritual place of Cardinal Joseph Bernadine, but I did try and accept that death wasn't my enemy.

One afternoon, after a particularly challenging day, Dr. DeMarco came into my room and pulled up a chair next to my bed. "Despite our most recent surgery, your heart continues to swell. Draining the excess fluid has helped, but it's still in really bad shape."

I was philosophical. "You know, in my classroom, I always tell my students to never forget who they are, never lose their identity or sense of themselves. I encourage them to learn their family history and deepen their faith, no matter what their tradition is. I push this each and every day to my class. I do it myself. I define myself every day. I am a man...I am a white man...I am a Catholic white man...I am a Catholic celibate white man...I am a heterosexual Catholic celibate white man.

"But if there is one thing this experience has taught me it's that all those titles and categories don't mean a damn thing because, according to you and the transplant team, I will likely lose my life within the next month or so, which means we are near the end of my journey in this life. At this point, you could give me a white heart, a black heart, a man's heart, a woman's heart, a Catholic heart, a Muslim heart, a Jewish heart, a gay heart, or a straight heart... if it's a human heart, and God wills it, and a family allows it, I will be grateful for the rest of my life. All those categories mean nothing when it's you that's on the gurney."

It was and is the greatest lesson of my life.

I would be very grateful to accept a human heart. Period. It didn't mean anything if the donor was a man or woman of a different faith, color, creed, or orientation. We have a shared humanity, and that is quite enough.

Never again would I limit myself by my own characteristics and categories. The possibility of my own death inspired me to see through how I limited myself. I have way more *in* common than *not* in common with all around me.

Perhaps, it was luck or simply good fortune—I'm convinced it was Divine Providence—but a few days after my talk with Dr. DeMarco, Bishop Wester stopped by for a visit. I had just given my brother and sister the bad news that despite the most recent surgery, my heart continued to swell 1 and I was still retaining fluids as my body weakened. By this time, I could no longer go for walks at night on the floor and had to limit my consumption of water because it was "too heavy" for my body. Instead, I was instructed to dine on ice chips and popsicles. It was pretty obvious we were running out of time.

My continued discipline of Centering Prayer kept me in a solid, grounded place. I knew the broken Jesus of the Cross was with me, but I was still a little nervous and scared as well. My brother and sister were praying for a miracle, while I was prepared to follow God's will, which meant a last bit of unfinished business.

"Bishop Wester, I think this might be a good time to anoint me…please. I sense we're getting close. I can't even walk anymore and I'm so drained, it's a struggle just getting out of bed to sit in a chair. I believe I'm ready."

I was requesting the Last Rites of the Catholic Church. I wanted to receive the sacrament while I was still sharp enough to appreciate the blessing. I didn't want to wait until it was too late. I also thought it would help Maureen and Johnny as they struggled in those dark moments. I could see the stress and tension on their faces. I knew the grace of the sacrament would help their spirits.

Bishop Wester said, "Joe, I would be honored to share this sacrament with you."

As Maureen and Johnny gathered around my bed, Bishop Wester began by saying, "Joe, Jesus is here. He is here now, in this room. Your mom and dad are here with you, and your sister and brother. Everyone who has visited throughout this difficult year is here—your students and faculty at Serra, all your friends, and those who have loved you all your life; they are all here."

And with that, he removed the sacred Oil of the Sick from the case he always carried and traced the sign of the cross on my forehead and my hands. "Joe, I anoint you with this Sacred Oil of the Church in Jesus name: the Father, Son, and Holy Spirit."

Next, he allowed my sister to dip her finger into the oil and bless me, and my brother followed. It was a beautiful moment. Maureen and Johnny added a few additional words of love and encouragement, and I felt love and faith all around me. I felt the spiritual presence of Mom and Dad, and I will forever be grateful to Bishop Wester for including my entire family in the anointing.

As a priest, I had anointed hundreds of people who were very sick or facing death, but I had never been anointed. I don't want to sound overdramatic, but something happened that night. I felt a peace come over me unlike anything I'd ever felt before. For the first time in a very long time, I knew...just absolutely knew that everything was going to be all right. I would be OK if I lived long enough to receive a transplant, and I would be fine if it didn't work out. I felt safe. I was centered in God's love and the love of my family and community.

For the first time in more than a year, I slept like a baby.

37

"Joe, we think we have a heart"

Days and nights on the 10th floor Cardiac Unit were long. Time stood still, and minutes felt like hours, and hours felt like days. For the most part, I lived on the 10th floor throughout 2005. I would come home from time to time, but I would either slip back into failure, or the defibrillator was would unleash its war cry and I would be on the floor dialing 911.

While prayer was important, so were the pastoral visits I received. One Friday night, after a particularly long day in which I began to cough up blood, a nurse came by and said there were several college-age young men standing in the hallway insisting that they needed to see Father Joe.

I recognized the voices and laughter and explained they were former students and would she please allow them in for a while, even though it was way past visiting hours. She smiled. "OK, Joe, but not for long."

When the door opened the kids, now young men, burst through with hugs and good cheer. It was fairly evident that the lads had visited one or more of San Francisco's finest establishments for adult refreshment before deciding to visit their old theology teacher. There is no such thing as a fun night on the 10th floor, since people literally are engaged in life and death struggles, but that night was the closest thing to it. The guys caught me up on all that was happening in their lives and the lives of their former high school classmates.

As the visit wound down, one of them asked if we could all pray together. It brought me back to prayer on the sideline of football games and joyful times in the classroom. We held hands, and the young men actually led the prayer, each offering their own insight and petition. I was overwhelmed with gratitude when they left because I realized there is no way anyone can survive on their own or just relying on private prayer. It is just not enough. There has to be a sense of community as well.

Every time I felt discouraged or lost, someone was there to offer support and encouragement. I received tons of prayer cards from people throughout the Archdiocese of San Francisco, many from those I didn't even know. It was deeply moving to read the cards and personal notes.

My name was added to prayer lists from different faith traditions. I received prayer cards from the local Episcopal Church, and one day, I received a "Message of Faith and Hope" from a Baptist Church in Atlanta, Georgia, who somehow learned of my plight from an online prayer tree. I don't know anyone from Atlanta, but I could sure feel their prayers during those long nights on the 10th floor. It was like the Lord was sending one angel after another to keep me centered and hopeful. And heart patients are a hopeful lot.

Just because someone is listed for a transplant doesn't mean they will receive it; it only means they need it. The sad truth is that many die waiting. I watched that happen at UCSF, and it was heartbreaking. My door was usually closed to prevent infection, but once in a while, I would peek out and see someone walking the hallways for some exercise. We would offer each other encouraging nods.

Then, after a while, I wouldn't see them, and I'd ask Dr. DeMarco what happened. They had become very sick, a few days would pass, and I'd ask a nurse or doctor if my walking pals were improving. Only then would I get the sad news that he or she had recently died. Sometimes, it was post-transplant rejection, and sometimes their body didn't hold out long enough to receive a new heart or lungs. What was especially tragic was that some of the patients who died were in and out of hospital *longer* than I was. That was hard to take, hard to accept, and I would pray for their surviving families.

Each day was largely the same. A staff member would enter my room about 5:00 AM to weigh me as a way to see if I was retaining more fluid, then an aid would check my legs and feet for additional signs of swelling. Usually, Dr. DeMarco or her associate, Dr. Dana McGlothlin, would come by around 10:00, followed closely by a group of interns, who often looked fresh out of high school, but were extremely knowledgeable about my condition. They were also not the least bit shy to offer additional comments and recommendations regarding my treatment. Later in the morning, I would receive an EKG, or electrocardiogram, in order to determine abnormal rhythms that put additional stress and tension on the heart muscle.

Because I didn't have the strength to get out of bed, I was relegated to lying still in the afternoon. My old partner from our Charlie's Angels days, Lynne Mullen, would bring up a laptop and we'd watch the latest DVDs...and watch the clock move to another day.

Then one afternoon, I met The Man, himself, the man who would actually do the transplant—the lead cardiac surgeon at UCSF, Dr. Charles Hoopes. If Dr. DeMarco and Dr. McGlothlin possessed warmth and hospitality, Dr. Charles Hoopes was an ice storm blowing across the unit. Their styles were as different as day and night.

My introductory meeting with Dr. Hoopes lasted all of thirty seconds, and I later learned it was quite an expansive conversation. In that short time span, he explained the severity of my condition and emphasized that I wouldn't go home until "we do this," and promptly whirled around and left the room.

I felt like Arnold Horshack in *Welcome Back Kotter* as I shouted, "Oh, oh, oh," in a futile effort to get the teacher's attention. I kept at it until I saw the door close. Still, he is a renowned transplant surgeon, and I felt blessed to have his expertise...even if our dialogue was always brief as humanly possible.

After he was gone, one of the transplant nurses walked over and, while dispensing medications, half-whispered with a hint of awe and fear, "So, you met him? You met Dr. Hoopes?"

"Yes, I believe I did. The warm, fuzzy guy who just flew out my room—that was him, right?"

The nurse laughed. "Yep, that was him. I'm afraid he doesn't have much of a bedside manner, but trust me, you want him doing your transplant. He is among the best in the world."

Dr. Hoopes not only performed the heart and lung transplant surgeries at UCSF, but he also performed heart valve repair and replacement surgery, often working with the most at-risk patients. I felt that if it ever happened, I had amazingly skilled and gifted doctors by my side in Dr. DeMarco and Dr. Hoopes.

If it ever happened.

And then, one day it did. It actually happened.

At 10:00 in the morning, August 5th, Dr. McGlothlin came in during her rounds to check on me, although this time she was alone. She calmly walked over to my bed and said, "Joe, we think we have a heart. Dr. Hoopes is in dialogue with another hospital, but it looks good. We should know for sure within the hour. I am so happy for you and your family."

I burst into tears. They tumbled down my face and landed on the sheets and pillows. My emotions came from such a deep place that my heart monitor actually began flying all over the place. "Easy Joe, I need you to stay calm. I know this is big, but I need you to calm down. Listen, you need to keep this to yourself because nothing is confirmed, OK? Just try and relax, don't say anything, and I will be back as soon as possible."

Dr. Dana McGlothlin had not walked into the hallway, when I violated every instruction she gave me. I reached for the phone and began calling anyone and everyone I had ever met in my entire life. I had my cell phone going and the phone next to the bed with two, sometimes three, conversations going on at the same time. I was so wrapped up in gratitude and joy that I lost track of who was on the other end.

It was an emotional call to Maureen and Johnny who dropped everything and headed to UCSF. I needed to collect myself before calling Bishop John Wester. He had been my rock among my brother priests. He was the one I could count on.

Bishop Wester, with calm sensitivity, prayed on the phone with me; it was a prayer for my donor and family, a prayer for the surgical team, and a prayer for the courage to accept God's will in the hours and days to come. He promised that he would offer Mass for the success of the surgery.

After our conversation, I took a moment to adjust my IV's, and removed the oxygen so I could slip out of bed and offer a prayer of thanksgiving to God.

This was my third gift.

The first was the grace to reclaim my faith. The second was the blessing of sobriety and ordination, and now, I was actually going to receive another one—a new heart.

Unbelievable.

Moments after I reconnected the IV's and oxygen and settled back into bed, Dr. McGlothlin reappeared with Dr. DeMarco. One look at Dr. D, and I exploded into tears again. She had walked with me through this journey from the first diagnosis to this moment. She had been there through some very dark days and had never given up on me. I mumbled an incoherent, "Thank you," as she offered up a big hug.

"We can do this," she whispered. "Try and relax, and I'll be back to check in with you later."

As both doctors walked to the door, Dr. McGlothlin paused and looked back, "Joe, it's OK now, go ahead and call your family and loved ones."

"Ah, gee, thank you…ah, I think I will." I'm sure my face turned beet red.

A short time later, Dr. DeMarco returned. "OK, Joe, we have tentatively scheduled you for transplant tonight at 8:00. I will be in to see you before then. In the meantime, try and get some rest. Tomorrow you will wake up to a whole new life. I'll see you in Recovery following your surgery. You're in good hands with Dr. Hoopes and his team."

My thoughts were consumed with my donor and family. Somewhere, someplace, a man or woman was being prepared to have their heart removed from their body and placed in mine. The mere thought of it was overwhelming. While a family grieved the loss of a loved one, someone made the decision to save my life by allowing the transplant to occur. I could not imagine the depth of generosity it took to make such an offer at a time of such profound loss.

I wondered about the soul of my donor. Did their soul rest in God, or was part of it living in me, since it was their heart keeping me alive? I decided I would never have a clear answer to such questions, since only God knows what happens to our soul. But I decided that since my donor's heart would live inside me, they would also be with me in a very spiritual way. Such a gift and blessing brought a spiritual dimension as well as physical.

The Transplant Unit at UCSF is a whirlwind of activity. There are patients waiting for their transplant, and there are those recovering from surgery—a recovery that can include moments of perilous rejection, where the body refuses to accept the new organ. It's a remarkable mix, each bringing its own unique set of physical, emotional, and spiritual challenges. The floor is intense 24/7, 365 days a year. Johnny once said that he could feel the intensity just driving into the parking lot.

The day of my surgery was no exception. At about 7:30 PM, a surgical nurse came into my room and announced that my transplant, originally scheduled for 8:00, was going to be pushed back until 10:00. She paused and followed by saying, "No problems at all, and everything is still a go."

I asked for anxiety medication and was given a valium; under the circumstances, it was entirely appropriate.

My room was filling up with extended family when the same surgical nurse came back in about 9:30 and said, "All is well, but we need to back you up to midnight. Try and relax, we're fine and I will be back."

About 11:30…you guessed it…the same nurse returned and said, "OK, this is what's going on; Dr. Hoopes and his team are completing a double lung transplant (I didn't know such a thing was possible.), and they want to take a little nap before bringing you down. So we will bring you down at 4:00AM and be ready to go."

No one said a word.

I broke the silence by saying, "Listen, you tell Dr. Hoopes to take all the time *he needs* because I need you sharp at 4:00 tomorrow morning."

The nurse laughed. "I'll be sure to pass on your instructions."

She returned at exactly 4:00AM. "OK, Joe, it's time, and we're ready."

I joined hands with my family and close friends, and several of the nurses came in to join us. After almost a year living on the floor, we were all on a first name basis. I felt their care, support, and love. We shared a nervous group hug, and it was time to go.

38

Surgery

Heart transplant surgery at UCSF is performed on the fourth floor. We all stepped into the elevator and went down together. I remember quietly humming the Entrance Hymn of my Ordination Mass, "Be Not Afraid."

As I signed off the final paperwork, a young nurse quietly emerged from a side room carrying a small igloo ice chest. I later learned that everyone else noticed the ice chest, too, and knew exactly what it contained. No one said a word, and neither did the nurse who stoically walked past my gurney and into the surgery room with my new heart literally in her hands.

A few moments later, the anesthesiologist appeared and explained that he was going to "give me something more to relax."

And that's the last thing I remember.

If everything goes perfectly, a heart transplant takes about seven hours. In understated layman terms, the surgeon makes an incision through the breast bone, and the patient's blood is then circulated through a heart and lung machine. At a certain point, the heart is removed from the body and the donor heart is placed inside and stitched into place. *If* the patient's body accepts the new organ and blood begins to flow from the transplanted heart, the heart-lung machine is removed and the patient begins breathing on his own.

Dr Hoopes and his team began my surgery around 4:30 in the morning, and they finished about 11:30—right on schedule. I found out later that everything went smoothly, and I was out of Recovery and in an ICU room by 1:00 PM. Absolutely amazing.

August 6th, 2005, became my new birthday.

When I woke up in the ICU, the first person I saw was my brother, Johnny. He was wearing a mask and whispering words of love and encouragement. "It's over; they did it, and you're doing great." He said it over and over again.

Dr. DeMarco had warned me that when I came to I would immediately notice the breathing tube down my throat and a multitude of IV's crisscrossed atop my body. I noticed them, all right, and they were a bit scary and uncomfortable. Thankfully, the doctors wanted me breathing on my own right away, so the breathing tube was quickly removed. The first day, I was encouraged to sit up and dangle my feet over the side of the bed. Other than the incision, I was pain-free.

The squeezing, tight pain that seemed to be always in my chest was no longer present, and when I took a deep breath, that terrible gurgling sound was gone as well. Hours before my surgery, Dr. DeMarco had told me that I wouldn't believe how great I'd feel afterward. As always, she was correct.

I took a peek at the scar down my chest and noticed an additional scar near my new heart—exactly where the defibrillator *used to be*. It had been removed during the surgery. No more shock therapy. If I hadn't been tethered to thirteen different IV lines, I would have jumped up and moonwalked across the room.

Dr. DeMarco came in for a quick exam. After listening to the steady beat of my new heart, she said, "That heart is way strong. Your surgery went perfectly, and you're on your way, Joe." Once again, I filled up with tears and was unable to speak. Dr. DeMarco gently patted my shoulder and was soon off to visit another patient.

As for Dr. Hoopes, I'm of the opinion that he must never sleep. Every time I woke up, he was standing next to the bed or pouring over charts outside my room. For the next forty-eight hours, he was never far from my room. Of course, staying true to form, he rarely spoke to me, but it was comforting knowing he was nearby.

Barely twenty-four hours post-transplant, I was encouraged to get out of bed and begin walking. I can't begin to describe the joy of walking again, since it had been months since I'd walked out of my room and strolled down the hallway. It was sheer heaven to feel my feet touch the hallway floor with my new heart beating steadily in my chest, and in perfect rhythm.

39

Post - Transplant

I found the physical recovery from heart transplant to be less taxing than several of the previous surgeries and procedures leading up to it. In fact, the biggest adjustment was more emotional than physical. I couldn't get over my good fortune. God and God's people have been extraordinarily good to me throughout my life, and there were times I betrayed such goodness. And now, I had received yet another blessing, another gift; I had a new, functioning heart, and was in the process of reclaiming my life.

The transplant team at UCSF is nothing if not thorough. They not only addressed the physical aspect of healing, but the emotional as well. Several days after the surgery, the social worker checked in with me. "Joe, you're beginning a new transition; you're moving from survival mode, where all thoughts and actions are focused on living long enough to experience transplant, to resuming and celebrating the reality of a new life. The transition won't happen overnight, so you have to be gentle with yourself and allow time to adjust."

Like all transplant patients, I rode an emotional roller coaster the first few days after surgery, and was focused on my donor and his or her family. I kept having this vision of another family grieving the loss of a loved one, while I celebrated another chance at life. I know it was impossible, but I wanted to reach out and console them.

I wondered if my donor was a man or woman. Did he or she have children? Did they die suddenly? Where did they live? The questions and feelings poured in from all angles, and at any time. One minute I thought I had pulled myself together, and the next I was crying my eyes out. I was told that my body was still in shock and was overloaded with steroids, and that was all part of getting through the process of recovery. But to be honest, I felt it went deeper than medications. It came from a place of gratitude that touched my soul.

As always during a difficult time, the good Lord sent yet another angel to help me. One afternoon, Dr. McGlothlin strolled into my room and found me balling my eyes out. I was on a roll, and the tears just wouldn't dry up. Some were tears of gratitude and some were tears of sorrow for my unknown donor and family. I couldn't tell the difference, they just kept pouring out.

Dr. McGlothlin calmly asked what was wrong. I babbled on about how I didn't deserve this sacrifice, I was most unworthy because of the mistakes I had made in my life. With typical patience that defines her approach to every medical dilemma, she said, "Joe, it's true that this gift can be overwhelming, but this heart now belongs to you. It is fully yours. The way you honor it is by taking great care of it. You aren't using someone else's heart; it has been given to you. You can show the depth of your gratitude by how you live with it. You wouldn't have received this new heart if your name hadn't come up as a match, but it did, and now you can move forward with your life and share this gift with others."

I looked directly at her and said, "I give you my word that I will live the rest of my life, one day at a time, with deep thanks for this blessing. And I will never forget what you and the whole team have done for me and my family. Thank you."

The following morning, the transplant coordinator, Celia Rifkin, stopped in to see me with some very basic news about my donor. He was a man in his 30s when he died, and she offered me a chance to write a general letter of thanksgiving to my donor's family.

I knelt on my knees and promised God that for the rest of my life I would begin each day with a prayer for my anonymous donor and his family.

That night, I began writing a letter to his family. I wasn't allowed to say anything about myself; it was to be a non-specific, brief letter of gratitude. It took me three days and nights and at least twenty-five drafts to find the right words. Finally, I realized that there were no "right" words, so I sat down and just poured out my feelings and prayers for his family. I sealed the letter and presented it to Celia. She smiled and promised to mail it that day.

I settled back in my chair, and gently touched my new heart. I couldn't believe how effortlessly it worked. It never missed a beat and felt strong and healthy. The doctors began encouraging me to walk at least twice a day, three if I could make it. Where I could barely move before, I was encouraged to be active.

Each day, my walks got a little longer and stronger, and more and more IV's were taken out of my body. I no longer needed oxygen to breathe, and was able to walk without assistance. I quickly began to feel like my old self again. Given the severity of this surgery, I was amazed at how fast and smoothly my recovery went. ·

Several days after surgery, I went back down to the 4th floor for my first biopsy. I walked into the surgical room and called out to the doctors and staff, "I know you all missed me, so I'm back for a quick visit. Yep, I can feel the love."

Although sedated, I could feel everything during the procedure. The surgeon goes back into my heart and actually takes a microscopic piece out from the base of my heart and runs it to the lab. Believe it or not, from this tiny piece, the doctors can tell how my body is adjusting to my new heart. I am constantly stunned at the brilliance of medical advances.

Later that afternoon, I learned there was evidence of moderate rejection, so they increased the steroids and rescheduled another biopsy in a few days. The following one went perfectly, and my new heart was said to be working beautifully. I even heard talk of going home.

After almost a year on and off the 10th floor, I was discharged from UCSF Medical Center, eleven days after my transplant. I was actually going home with a new heart. The day before I was released, Dr. DeMarco came in and said, "If you can walk around the halls of the 10th floor three times, I think you'll be ready to go home."

Bolstered with the challenge, I grabbed the arm of my old friend, Lynne Mullen, who was visiting, and said, "Let's go."

I wouldn't call it a jog, or even a fast walk, but we made it three times around the entire area. I stopped by a few rooms to offer encouragement to patients waiting for their miracle, and I also stopped to thank the remarkable nurses who took care of me during the long year.

The morning I was set to go home, Dr. Hoopes stopped by. I literally grabbed his arm, and held on before he could make his usual speedy retreat. Not this time, Doc. "You saved my life, Dr. Hoopes. Your skill as a surgeon has given me another chance at life, and I am so grateful to you. My family is so grateful to you. I want you to know that I will treasure and honor my new heart forever. Thank you for the amazing care you and the staff gave me."

I only stopped because the tears of joy made it impossible to continue. I stood and hugged him. Dr. Hoopes responded in typical fashion, "There were a lot of people involved in your care. You go on now and live your life…but I will see you in clinic next week."

And with that he pulled away and disappeared down the hallway to visit another patient.

The Fourth Gift:
New Life

40

A New Beginning

One of the first lessons you learn as a heart transplant patient is the day of your surgery is not the *end* of your journey, it is the *beginning*.

I visited the Transplant Clinic each day for the first month I was home. Since I was not allowed to drive for the first six weeks, my transplant was, once again, a community effort. Five days a week, a variety of people offered to drive me into the city for additional treatments and biopsy tests to measure for signs of rejection.

Like all transplant patients, I take several anti-rejection medications throughout the day, and I will take them every day for the rest of my life. No big deal when one considers the alternative. The meds have side effects, but that's no big deal, either. None of it can compare to sitting day after day on the 10th floor not knowing if I was going to live or die. To this day, I have never missed one of my scheduled meds—I owe it to my donor and the transplant team.

I was taught that, oddly enough, my body would actually like to reclaim my old heart. It actually prefers the old one, and considers my new heart a foreign object. At any time, it is ready to attack the new heart because my body considers it a threat to my system. Thus, the whole point of the anti-rejection medications is to keep my immune system at a very low level so it doesn't attack my new heart. Taking the meds is not an option for transplant patients.

Here is the medication schedule I received the first week post-transplant, which covers the basic meds a transplant patient consumes on a daily basis. Of course, there are variations depending on the patient, but I think this passes for the primary schedule:

1. Cellcept: 750 mg. 2 times per day—prevent rejection
2. Prograff: 2 mg. 2 times per day—prevent rejection
3. Valcyte: 450mg. 2 times per day—anti viral; prevent infection
4. Potassiom: 250mg. 4 times per day—important mineral for cell function
5. Furosemide: 40 mg. 1 time per day—reduce swelling and fluid retention
6. Diovan: 180mg. 1 per day—treatment of high blood pressure
7. Norvasc: 20 mg. 1 time per day—treatment of high blood pressure
8. Prednisone: 60 mg. 1 time per day—immunosuppresent (later reduced)
9. Topril: 300 mg. 1 per day—treatment for high blood pressure
10. Calcium: 250mg. 1 per day — mineral supplement
11. Septra: 400mg. M/W/F — antibiotic to prevent infection
12. Glipizide: 5mg. 1 per day — anti diabetic treatment
13. Lipitor: 40 mg 1 per day — treat high cholesterol

There you have it. Nothing to it. When I came home, I posted a spread sheet on the fridge and checked off meds each day. After a while, it became part of my routine.

The problem with maintaining a low immune system is it makes you vulnerable to colds and infections. During my first year, I picked up a minor cold and, before I knew it, I was back in UC with pneumonia. There was nothing to stop the virus from working its way through my system. Thus, a transplant patient has to be incredibly careful to avoid routine colds and infections, since they can lead to serious problems.

In fact, the first three years post-transplant, I averaged at least one hospital visit each year. It was almost always a cold or flu bug that worked its way into pneumonia. I would call in the symptoms and return to the 10th floor for treatment. I was usually home within the week.

I often relate my transplant to living life as a sober priest. I can never afford to take it for granted, but it has changed and enriched my life beyond all imagining.

41

Seeking Reinstatement as a Priest

It took several months to get used to having a new heart. A transplanted heart beats faster than a normal heart, and it took some time to realize that the faster beat was the new normal for me. But all said, my recovery went remarkably well and was reasonably painless. I checked in daily, then weekly, and then monthly with Dr. DeMarco. Within six months, I felt good enough to ask her about returning part-time to my life as a priest. I missed not being in a parish or part of a school community.

We agreed to begin slow and see how things progressed. Dr. DeMarco said, "I'm all in favor of your return to ministry, but you need to remember that you have physical risks. You will always need to be extremely careful not to pick up your basic cold because it can and will cause major problems for you. So you need to take every precaution necessary to remain healthy."

I would undergo monthly blood tests to check how my body was reacting to the anti-rejection meds. Nothing was left to chance, and Dr. DeMarco gave me full clearance to return to my life as a priest on a part-time basis.

When a priest has been permitted a leave of absence, he must receive approval from a Bishop and the personnel board before beginning a new assignment. Six months after my transplant, my first order of business was to set an appointment with the Bishop. Sitting in his office, I told him that I had learned a lot during the past year— about life, and death, and dealing with a serious illness. "Bishop Wester, I'm living proof that God intervenes in the darkness. The fact that I am alive, clean and sober, and walking around with a new heart is testimony to His love—to say nothing of His *remarkable* patience. By all rights, I should be dead. I could have died with Steve that terrible day, I could have died in various car accidents in the years to follow, I could have died using dangerous drugs my first year at St. Joseph's, and I could have died on the transplant table…but for some reason I didn't. I honestly believe God kept me alive for a specific purpose. I don't think this just *happened*. God was in control and saved me to help with His work. That has to be it—I can't think of any other reason. Can you?"

Bishop Wester smiled. "No, my friend, I believe God has a plan for you. Tell me what you want to do and where you would like to go."

"Bishop, I believe God saved me to share my story. Fr. Bob Gavin told me that my first year at St. Patrick's, but I'm not sure I believed him. I thought I was unworthy. And maybe I still am, but God isn't. I'm alive to share this with others so they can learn from my mistakes and see that some problems are too much for us, but not when we place our faith in God and a supportive community. I want—hell, I *need* to preach the importance of both."

We talked about my eventual return to Serra to serve part time as chaplain, but in the meantime he suggested I move into St. Gregory's Parish to serve on a part-time basis. The pastor, Msgr. Robert McElroy, who was soon to become Bishop McElroy, welcomed me to St. Gregory's, where I have continued to live ever since.

42

A New Mission and Ministry

When I arrived at St. Gregory's Parish, I hit the ground running. A new heart has a dramatic way of affecting how one looks at time. I greeted every day as a pure blessing, so I didn't want to waste any of it.

Lars Lund, who replaced me as president of Serra High School, invited me back for Mass with the entire school. It was extremely emotional for me because the faculty, students, former students, and staff had offered tremendous support in the months leading to my transplant. Now, I had a wonderful opportunity to thank them and celebrate Mass as our way to thank God for the grace of a new heart and the chance to come home.

During the homily, I told the students that the guidelines for having a heart transplant are very strict and rigorously enforced, and no one is ever allowed to cut corners. To even qualify, I had to have the same size heart as my donor—I'm a big guy, so a tiny heart would never work. In addition, we had to share the same blood type, and a host of tissue samples all had to match perfectly. If each and every part matched just right, then it is possible to proceed.

I looked into the young faces of the students and said, "Consider the odds against it. How likely is it that all those factors will match? Not at all, and it's why so many people die while waiting for a transplant. I actually have a photo of my donor that I keep in my room. If you saw him, you would see that we don't look alike, we aren't the same color, we aren't the same age, we don't live in the same area, or go to the same schools. We *look* so different, and we *are* so different, yet his heart is a perfect match for mine. His heart beats for me. His heart lives inside of me, giving me new life. His heart allows me to be here to thank you for all your support. Never think that we aren't brothers and sisters under God...I am here to tell you that we most certainly are.

"Believe me, when it's your butt on the gurney and your life is flashing before you, you won't care what heart you receive. Black or white, man or woman, gay or straight, it won't make a damn bit of difference—as long as it's a human heart, you will hit your knees in gratitude.

"We waste so much time, alienating ourselves from each other. We waste so much time fighting over our differences, but all that fades into nothing when you are desperate to reclaim your health and your life. Trust me, you will actively seek hope, and pray to find that which we share and have in common."

My message definitely resonated with the community, which was a wonderful mix of faith and ethnicity. My message was simple and direct; it was just one of the messages I learned from the previous year: In the end, we are the same.

43

A New Priest

I think when you combine the gift of sobriety and the blessing of a heart transplant into one life, you should emerge, you *must* emerge, somewhat different. I think both gifts changed my perspectives on life and my ministry as a priest.

Because I didn't have a spiritual answer to solve my own dilemma of needing a new heart, I stopped trying to provide simple answers for the complex problems people face while struggling through serious illness. Gone are the days when I would walk into a hospital setting and suggest an answer to a patient's dilemma as if I had direct knowledge from on high. It's just not that simple.

Illnesses are messy. They don't conform to any set standard. My year at UCSF Medical Center humbled me to that fact, and it was an important lesson for my life as a priest.

Today, I try to walk the path *with* the person, much as Bishop Wester walked it with me. I walk with clear eyes and an open heart, seeking only to be there for the patient. I give them room to work through problems on their own without interference from me. My goal is to serve more as a guide, someone to talk with during those scary moments we all face while in the hospital. I listen more and talk less—always a major challenge throughout my life. As a patient, I learned that people want their minister to listen rather than overwhelm them with solutions.

Although he has been gone for many years, I still remember the advice Fr. Bob Gavin gave me in the days leading up to my ordination (it only took twenty-one years to understand what he meant). His advice was, "Joey, never underestimate the ministry of presence."

"Ministry of presence? What do you mean?"

"It means to be there for your people—physically, emotionally, and spiritually; it doesn't mean that you always have an answer ready and prepared, it just means you are very present to whoever calls on you. You are there willingly, and completely focused on their needs. Don't worry about what to say, and don't worry whether you have the perfect answer to every problem they face. None of that is as important as establishing trust that you are completely present to whatever the person is going through."

Today, clean and sober, and strolling about with a new and healthy heart, I get it. I understand what my mentor was trying to teach me. My role is not to provide all the answers—only God can do that. My role is to walk the path, walk the journey with the person as they find their own way to God.

And that is what I try and do now as a priest. I do listen more and talk less. I try to really hear what he or she is saying and feeling. I don't stroll into a hospital room dispensing expertise on what a person should do or feel. I gently enter the sanctuary of their suffering and quietly listen. I try and become a quiet presence that walks with them through their darkness.

The approach has made a huge difference in my ministry. When I visit patients in the hospital, I no longer limit my visits to patients who are Catholic. I figure if I was more than willing to receive a Protestant, or Jewish, or Muslim heart, the least I can do is visit them when they are sick. Frankly, religious affiliation is no longer relevant for my time or visits. Since I never questioned the religious affiliation of someone who came to visit me, I think I'm quite fine to extend a prayer to anyone who welcomes me into their hospital room.

As a newly ordained priest, I used to show up at the front desk of a hospital and ask the receptionist for the list of Catholic patients who asked for a visit. Not anymore. Today, I still get my list, but when I'm finished with those visits, I will usually just walk the floor. If anyone sees me from their bed and calls me in…well, I am there. I owe it to the people who stopped in to visit me.

Recently, I was at UCSF and walked through the 10th floor to visit patients waiting for a transplant, or in recovery from their surgery. I saw a man sitting in a chair with a forlorn look that spoke of utter despair. His look reminded me of those last weeks before my transplant.

I waved at him and invited myself in. "Hey, I know how you're feeling. If you want to talk, I'm here."

"Yeah, Father, that's what they all say."

"No, man, you don't understand. This is room 1024… my old room…and I spent almost a year living here."

His eyes lit up. "Did you have a transplant?"

"Yep, and I rode the same roller coaster you're on."

"Pull up a chair, Father, thanks for stopping by."

It made all the difference — for both of us. I sat and listened to his worries about his family, his financial concerns, and his spiritual fears. In the end, he asked for my blessing, and I asked for his.

I remember his surprise, "What, I've never blessed a priest before."

"Well, its time you did, because we are facing the same struggles; how about we bless and then pray for each other. We are both doing the best we can with what we've got."

We both prayed silently for each other, and felt the shared spirit.

Sobriety and my transplant have humbled my ministry. And I am so very grateful.

44

My New Life

There is a great story about St. Francis of Assisi. It seems that before sending his Friars out on mission, he would gather them together and offer some simple, but challenging advice: "Preach the Gospel at all times. If necessary, use words."

My journey from drug and alcohol use to sobriety has been a journey to finally live what I preach. As a functioning alcoholic I rarely did. I would say the right things, but that was all part of the game, especially that first year in seminary. I would do whatever I wanted. My talk and actions were often miles apart. The blessing of sobriety changed all that because I don't believe anyone can live a sober life without unconditional honesty.

That is the whole point of working the steps to recovery; it forces you to confront yourself. The days of hiding and shading the truth for my own benefit were over. Thank God.

I once heard a person at a meeting say, "You just can't function with a head full of A.A. and a belly full of beer."

Amen.

Today, I devote a major part of my ministry to sharing my story because it's my humble hope that it can touch someone and show that there really is another way. Once after speaking at a Catholic college campus, a student came up afterward and asked, "Father Joe, what is the best thing about sobriety? What are you most grateful for?"

The answer was easy. "The best part, the part for which I am most grateful, is simply being able to wake up in the morning and look myself in the mirror. There were years when I couldn't do it because I was so ashamed. I love to wake up sober and look at myself, and know I have no more regrets. It is an absolute blessing."

Sobriety taught me how to pray. I will never forget Fr. Bob telling me that he saw my drinking and using as a "grace." Now, almost twenty-six years later, I know what he meant. It gave me the humility to crawl back to God. I didn't walk into the chapel to seek forgiveness and healing, I crawled to it. The game was up and I had no defenses left. I had reached my official bottom. Sitting on a chair in a Catholic seminary chopping up methamphetamine was my official bottom.

I thought entering the seminary would be a major step forward in my life, and I turned it into a huge step backward. After castigating myself as the single greatest fraud to ever enter a religious house, I *still used it*, and finally *accepted* that I was in way over my head and something was very wrong. I finally had the absolute grace to realize that I simply could not stop. I might have wanted to stop, but I couldn't. It had become part of who I was.

For me, there was always a big difference between *feeling* I had a problem and *accepting* I had a problem. I could "feel" it all day and it didn't really matter because I just kept going. But "accepting" it was a whole different ballgame.

I learned to trust the mysterious workings of the Lord, and I learned to trust in His people. God and community worked together to save me from a life of drinking and using, and I just knew they would see me through the process to transplant…whether I actually received a new heart or not.

Without faith and the love of my family, extended family, and supportive community, I never would have made it.

It was too much to handle alone. For me, the mountain was too high to climb and fell on my own too many times. I needed God in my life. I needed sober people in my life.

Together they saved me.

45

Warning from Brother Priests

I began jotting down some thoughts and ideas for this memoir about three years ago after I wrote an article for the *San Francisco Catholic Newspaper* about my experience of receiving a heart transplant. It led to several friends encouraging me to write a memoir that included the spiritual journey to sobriety.

It had to be completely honest, but not at the risk of hurting anyone else. That is why, unless I received explicit permission, I refrained from sharing names of people who shared elements of the journey with me.

After completing an early manuscript, I showed it to a priest I trust and respect. He returned it to me a few days later with a cautionary word: "Joe, be very careful with this. Although I know the truth of your story, this is going to shock people...they might be angry and turn on you...this is too dangerous...I would hold back on some of the details."

I thanked him for sharing, and quickly turned to someone else for one more take. His response was a bit more firm. "You cannot write about using drugs in the seminary. No, you just cannot do that. This will be a scandal."

I responded, "Look, I didn't share it for dramatic effect; I wrote it because it was true. I violated the rules because I was in way over my head, and the 'fault' belongs to no one but me. The reason I wrote this is to show that there is another way to live and you can work yourself out of addictions, so long as you have faith in God and support from God's people. I believe this is a hopeful book."

He answered with a much stronger voice. "Joe, don't you see? People see us in a different light than they see other people in their community. They don't want to hear about a past that included drinking and drug use. You can share this at your meetings and support groups, but it won't play well with church-going folks. There is no way this should be published in its present form."

So, true to form, I responded with a voice (just slightly) elevated. "But the story is true, dammit. What's the problem with sharing the truth when it might touch someone else and help them through a challenging time? My recovery is based on honest sharing of past mistakes so others may benefit. There is no hidden agenda here—it's the story of how one priest was literally saved from himself…twice. Once by way of sobriety, and the other by organ transplant."

He responded with equal elevation: "I think this will just cause trouble that we don't need. No one wants to hear about out-of-control drinking and drug use on the way to becoming a priest. I can't support this."

I ended the dialogue. "I feel for you, man, I really do. I'm not afraid of the truth, but you are."

And that was the last time I asked one of my brothers if I should write this memoir. Let's just say we agreed to disagree.

Deep down, I understood the concern. For at least two decades, the priesthood has been devastated by horrific stories of abuse and covering up the sins of its own priests. By doing so, it has done incalculable harm and damage to families. Of course, the fallout has been that we have lost much of our credibility with a significant number of our flock. No one can doubt or question that as fact.

I think as hurt and angry people as were about the crimes committed against children and young people, they were equally angry about the systematic cover up by the Church hierarchy. They placed the preservation of their own reputation before the righteous healing of the victims.

In light of such of such deception, what can possibly be wrong with sharing an honest story of recovery—one that includes spiritual, emotional, and physical rehabilitation? Why continuously run from the truth? Why pretend something is true when it isn't?

I suppose my brothers might be more comfortable with a story of a young man who grew up in a wonderful family and entered the seminary where he went on to become a solid and dependable priest. Well, I did grow up in a wonderful family, but it is equally true that due to an inability to handle emotional loss and grief, I drank and used everything under the sun...even while I was a seminarian.

I believe I experienced two miracles in my life. No one can ever tell me that my sobriety and the blessing of a new heart were not totally connected to God. I also believe that I was saved so I could share my story to help others. The price of trust is honesty, regardless of our comfort and reputation.

When I was in high school, I looked up to our priests, and a major reason was because they were honest with us. Fr. John Kelly never shied away from a challenging truth, and that touched me in such a way that I wanted to become what he was—a Catholic priest. He never hid from the truth or ducked away from challenging issues concerning the Church. He influenced an entire generation of students because of his honesty and willingness to confront issues that affected us.

I hope this story has, in some small way, inspired you to see that there really is a way out of addiction, and there really is hope in the midst of a life threatening disease like heart failure. I also hope I have not hurt anyone with the facts of my story. Please know that was never my intention. The mistakes were mine, and I take full responsibility.

Priests are *not* different from anyone else, and they should not be treated or looked at differently. We are capable of wonderful acts of charity and healing, and we are capable of falling into addictions and needing treatment for a failing heart. This book is an attempt to tell a true story that has a grace-filled ending...and a new beginning.

I don't want to hide from it or pretend it doesn't exist. I would rather use it to help someone else.

46
For An Old Friend

Several years ago, I concelebrated a Mass for a man I knew well from our school days as youngsters. In the world of elementary school romance, he was a major hit with the girls and set the standard for all the boys to follow. He had girls flocking to him without even trying. Boys like me were envious of his skill on the playground. He was also the fastest kid in the class, which meant he had the respect of our adult coaches as well. He was a home run everywhere he went.

I remember smoking marijuana and drinking with him in high school and in the years that followed. He remained the same funny and popular guy he'd always been. One night we bumped into each other at a local pub and held court for several hours. Like me, he was in way over his head with alcohol, but hadn't accepted it. In fact, for years to come, he refused to accept he had a problem.

We lost touch when I moved on to the airlines and seminary, but from time to time I would hear things about him that really concerned me. He was living at home as something of a recluse, but each day he would emerge around noon and walk to the local liquor store to purchase alcohol. He would spend most of the day watching TV and drinking, and living like a hermit. Now that is a long fall from someone who controlled a room just by walking through the door.

I saw him once more. He was standing outside a supermarket asking for change. We were in our thirties, and I was already a priest, working on my own sobriety. He recognized me and we chatted at great length. I told him of my battle for sobriety and new concern regarding my heart. Interestingly, he wouldn't look at me when I mentioned sobriety, but when I talked about a possible heart transplant he came to life. He was my old friend again. Funny, caring, concerned, and totally centered on the other person.

I realize now that he couldn't talk about sobriety because he felt it was so far past him, so he avoided talking about it, even with old friends like me. I embraced him as we parted ways and slipped him a few dollars, even though I knew where it would go. I left feeling helpless and sad.

It was only a year later when I received a call that he had died after a night of drinking and watching TV in his childhood home. I concelebrated his funeral Mass, and afterwards went to lunch with some mutual friends. A close friend of his shook her head, "We tried, we tried, we tried; it's just such a heartbreaking waste of a life."

"Waste of a life." Her words haunted me. He was a friend and a very gentle man who never hurt anyone—he wasn't capable of hurting anyone—and yet he died alone with nothing and no one around him. He only hurt himself.

I wrote this book for my old friend. I wish I had stayed and shared stories from this book. I wish we had talked longer. It's too late now, but maybe not for someone else. I wrote this for people like me who could have suffered the same fate. I wrote the story because it is true and, with all humility, too important not to share.

So if this book in anyway tarnishes my reputation as a priest, I am willing to take the heat. If what I've shared rocks anyone's image of priesthood and seminary, please blame me because the choices I made were mine. The priests in this book are blameless for how I chose to live back in the day; that is, until the grace of God touched me. His people helped save me.

Thank you for reading my story, I hope in some small way, it helped someone. There really is another way.

God, Grant me the *Serenity* to accept the things I cannot change,
The *Courage* to change the things I can.
And the *Wisdom* to know the difference.
One day at a time.
With Gratitude,
Fr. Joe

Acknowledgments

Mom and Dad, thank you for the gift of faith. While writing sections, especially early in the book, I could sense and almost see Mom in heaven shaking her head at some of my language. Sorry, Mom, it won't happen again. Promise.

Maureen and Johnny, thank you for being the greatest brother and sister in the world. I love you both, and I am so very grateful for you love and patience.

Brian and Diana, thank you for your wonderful and amazing support. I am very grateful.

My nieces and nephews: I hope I haven't disappointed you with this book. I am so grateful for all your support when I was sick. Thanks, Megan, Kevin, JT, Brittany, and Adrianna.

Dr. DeMarco, you saved my life. Thank you for all you did for me and my family. I will never forget your time and patience during some really dark days.

Dr. McGlothli, I am so grateful for your willingness to talk and encourage me. Thank you, from my entire family.

Dr. Charles Hoopes, I guess there is no point seeking to engage in a long conversation. But please know of my profound gratitude. I was so blessed to have you as my transplant surgeon. You gave me my life back. Thank you.

UCS, thank you to the doctors, nurses, and staff for your tireless devotion. I keep you in my prayers always and thank you for all you do.

I am grateful to Fr. Joseph Girzone and Fr. Adam Forno for their willingness to help and support a nervous and stumbling first time writer. Special thanks to Maria Fassio

Pignati for your encouragement and willingness to read through an early draft.

I am grateful to members of the staff at St. Gregory's Parish for reading several drafts and offering insight: Karen Elmore, Paula Ceccoti, Lorraine Paul, and Donna DeBenedetti—a great friend, even if you taught at St. Ignatius. Thank you.

Thank you to Lars Lund and Barry Thornton for your encouragement and support.

Thank you to Peggy Farrell, Patty Ferretti, and Patrick Walsh for your willingness to read early drafts.

Thank you to Chuck and Lucy Fontenot. You were there for all of it. Thanks, Kari, for your prayers. I have absolutely no doubt that David's spirit was with me on the 10th floor of UCSF. Thank you, David.

Thanks to Terrie Peterson and Kenny Romes, friends to Steve Olsen and me. Thank you for being there as this project came together.

Thank you to the Olsen family. Your son and brother was my friend. Steve has always been part of my life. Thank you for allowing me to share our story.

Thank you to Lynne Kennedy Mullen, my walking partner on the 10th floor. Your prayers and support helped in so many ways; thank you.

A special word of thanks to Fr. Bob Gavin—I love you Fr. Bob. You saved my spiritual life. I think of you often and feel so blessed to have known you at a critical time in my life.

Thank you to Msgr. Bruce Dreier and Fr, Jerry Coleman for being remarkable examples of priesthood.

Thank you, John Kelly, for being John Kelly.

Thank you, Fr. John Ryan, for being a friend and mentor throughout my life as a priest.

Charlie's Angels: You Rock. Thank you for blessing me with your goodness.

And to the man, who literally walked the journey with me, Bishop John Wester. *You* are a true shepherd. You shine the light of hope, the light of Jesus, on all you meet. My family and I thank you for your gentle presence to us. God's people are blessed by your faith and service. Thank you from the bottom of my new heart.

And finally, and most importantly, to Claire Gerus, my agent. Thank you, Claire. You believed in this project from the very beginning and offered wisdom and encouragement throughout. I am profoundly grateful.

Thank you Lynn Price, who published our book. Thank you, Lynn, for giving a first-time writer an opportunity to share his story. I am grateful for your generous time and belief in me.

Thank you Kathleen Murray Lynch, for your editing skills and faith in this project.

And to Jesus of the Cross: I thank you for my Four Gifts…my faith, my sobriety, my new heart, and my new life. They are mine, but they belong to You.